Internet Cool Tools for Physicians

Melissa L. Rethlefsen · David L. Rothman · Daniel S. Mojon

Internet Cool Tools
for Physicians

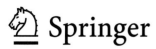 Springer

Melissa L. Rethlefsen
Learning Resource Center
Mayo Clinic Libraries
200 First St SW
Rochester, MN 55905
USA

David L. Rothman
Information Services Specialist
Community General Hospital
Medical Library
4900 Broad Rd
Syracuse, NY 13215
USA

**Prof. Dr. med. Daniel S. Mojon, MD,
FEBO, Exec. MHSA**
Head, Department of Strabismology
& Neuro-Ophthalmology
Kantonsspital St. Gallen
Rorschacher Strasse 95
9007 St. Gallen
Switzerland

ISBN: 978-3-540-76381-9   e-ISBN: 978-3-540-76382-6

Library of Congress Control Number: 2008933854

© 2009 Springer-Verlag Berlin Heidelberg

Cover design: Frido Steinen-Broo, eStudio Calamar, Spain
Cover picture: Prof. Dr. Daniel Mojon, Kantonsspital St. Gallen, Switzerland

Printed on acid-free paper

9 8 7 6 5 4 3 2 1

springer.com

Acknowledgments

Thanks to Colin Segovis for inspiration and help,
and to Elizabeth Fowler for her support and patience

Contents

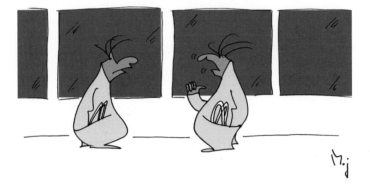

Introduction

As the single most powerful information tool in history, the Internet has changed everything and has only just begun changing the practice of medicine. Fortunately, the individual physician can also leverage the power of the Net to his or her own individual circumstances and needs. No single book will turn a physician into an Internet expert, but this one offers the savvy physician a large handful of shortcuts to getting to most out of free Internet tools and tricks. Leveraged intelligently, these can save the physician time, money, and hassle.

Personalized Web pages, RSS, social networks, social bookmarking, and note-taking tools can help make manageable the constantly growing avalanche of new information (both clinical and nonclinical) that the busy physician must assimilate.

Knowing what search tool to use for what sort of information and tricks for using each search tool effectively can save your valuable time when you know exactly what you're looking for and don't want to waste time sorting through irrelevant search results.

Podcasts, vodcasts, blogs, and wikis can serve not only as useful information resources to physicians, but also along with online collaboration tools, they provide physicians with an opportunity which is genuinely new in the history of health information. That opportunity is the fact that it is now within the budget and technological skills of virtually any doctor to become not only a discerning consumer of online health information but also a creator of healthcare information.

The Web will continue to evolve, and patients will continue to use it for seeking information about their health concerns and about their healthcare providers. Recent studies disclose that more than 70% of patients have been influenced by online health information in their treatment decision. However, the task of finding high-quality, appropriate health information can be an arduous process. Incomplete and misleading information may directly harm patients by misdirecting a treatment decision. Therefore, the dialogue between the physician and patient about Internet-based health information is getting more and more important. Besides, patients increasingly expect that their physicians can be reached through the Internet. These are all good reasons to keep up with Internet developments and to read this book.

1.1
What's the Future of the Internet?

Nobody knows exactly what the Internet or the Web will look like in the future. Once, PCs were the primary way to connect to the Internet. Now,

M. Rethlefsen et al., *Internet Cool Tools for Physicians*
© Springer-Verlag Berlin Heidelberg 2009

Internet-enabled devices such as pocket-sized PDAs and cell phones allow mobile access from nearly anywhere. This is a step toward global wireless communication.

Another key trend is that of the intelligent Web, an online channel is working for you. Not that data will become intelligent (most likely computer networks will never be able to reproduce human intelligence), but, instead, that data will be used more intelligently by humans. Web sites and social networking applications will allow physicians to aggregate relevant medical information to their level of experience and identify knowledge gaps. High-speed networks will increasingly allow physicians around the world to share specialized knowledge. Web-based consultations, diagnoses, and surgery will provide remote healthcare to astronauts on extended space journeys. And who knows, while reading a future edition of this book, your Internet-enabled GPS watch will warn you to move because the trajectory of a falling object will soon cross your position.

1.2
Glossary

For most of the terms we'll be using throughout this book, we'll provide definitions in the text. Before we even begin talking about Internet Cool Tools, however, it will help you to have some terms firmly in hand. Thus, we're providing this brief glossary to help you along your Cool Tools journey.

Internet. The Internet is a network connecting computers together globally. Any computer can communicate with any other computer as long as they are both connected to the Internet. Information travels over this network by a variety of languages known as *protocols*, including protocols for email and for the World Wide Web.

World Wide Web or Web. The World Wide Web, or briefly Web, is a way of accessing informa-

tion over the Internet. It utilizes browsers, such as Internet Explorer or Firefox, to access Web documents called *Web pages* that are linked to each other via hyperlinks. Web documents may contain text, graphics, sounds, and video. The Web uses a protocol called *hypertext transfer protocol* (HTTP) to transmit data. However, it is just one way that information can be disseminated over the Internet. The majority of tools that we discuss in this book are Web-based.

Link. A link, or hyperlink, is a connection between two documents on the Web. By clicking on a link, your Web browser will take you to a different Web page or a different location in the Web page you are using.

URL. URL is short for uniform resource locator and is also commonly known as a *Web address*. A URL works just like a postal address – a set of instructions telling you how to get to a location – but instead of a physical location, a URL takes you to a location on the Web. Like a physical address, there is only one URL for any given document on the Web – there are no duplicate addresses.

Browser or Web browser. A browser or Web browser is the piece of software you use to access the data on the Web. To see Web content, you must use a browser – it's basically your interpreter. Common browsers include Internet Explorer, Mozilla Firefox, Safari, and Opera, though of these, Internet Explorer is by far the most common. Web browsers are also often built into Web-accessible phones like the BlackBerry, the iPhone, and others.

Firefox. Mozilla Firefox is a freely available Web browser. You can download it at http://www.mozilla.com/firefox/. What's different about Firefox is that it is highly customizable. Firefox users can add extensions, or add-ons, to their Firefox browser to make it behave exactly like they want. Browser extensions may customize the look and feel of the browser or may get as fancy as changing how certain Web sites operate.

Occasionally throughout this book, we'll be referring to various Firefox add-ons and tools available only for Firefox users. We highly recommend using Firefox as your primary browser.

Internet Explorer. Internet Explorer is the most commonly used Web browser, primarily because it comes packaged with Microsoft operating systems. Newer versions of Internet Explorer have greatly improved the functionality of this tool, making it more like Firefox. Version 7+ even includes built-in tools like a new RSS reader (see Chap. 11) and tabbed browsing.

Bookmark. What is called a bookmark in Firefox and other browsers is called a *favorite* in Internet Explorer. They are equivalent terms describing marking a Web page for later retrieval. Browser-based bookmarks are stored in Bookmarks or Favorites folders.

Bookmarklet. Bookmarklets are small pieces of code that you add to your browser just like a bookmark. Instead of taking you to a new Web site, however, bookmarklets may perform other actions. In a few spots in this book, we'll be talking about a few tools that use bookmarklets to help you connect with their services.

Toolbar. In every browser, there is usually the standard toolbar with the location bar (where the Web page URL appears), a home icon to take you to your home page, stop and refresh buttons, and so on. You can install additional toolbars in your browser to soup it up. We will be discussing several useful toolbars in this book.

Web 2.0. Web 2.0 is a piece of jargon that we won't be using in this book, but which you might hear in reference to many of the Cool Tools we're covering. Essentially, Web 2.0 refers to a set of principles that has come to define Web sites after the dot com bust. These principles include some technical components, but the main focus is on participation. This second generation of dynamic Web-based services and communication tools allows all Web users to create and share content easily. Information sharing, notably through collaboration between users, and creativity are making the Web a hotbed for new and exciting content. New terms (most of which we'll be covering in this book) emerging with the Web 2.0 include tagging and folksonomies, feeds, mashups, blogs, wikis, podcasts, and vodcasts.

Social software. Social software simply means Web sites and tools that enable communication and sharing. The majority of tools that we cover in this book are considered social software. Other terms occasionally used interchangeably with social software include social media and social networking software, though social software is the broader term.

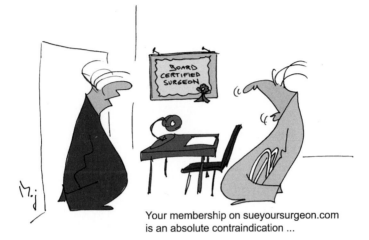

Your membership on sueyoursurgeon.com
is an absolute contraindication ...

Core Messages

- › Every search engine searches different and rarely overlapping content from the Web.
- › When you use a search engine, you aren't searching the "live" Web, just that particular search engine's snapshot of what is in its own database of Web content.
- › Google is the most popular search engine in most countries because of its highly relevant results.
- › Take advantage of Google's built-in features to make your searching even better.

2.1
Google

Though other search engines are also excellent for finding information, Google is the most popular search engine in almost every country outside of Southeast Asia. Known for its easy to use interface and highly relevant results, Google also places heavy emphasis on helping consumers and medical professionals find high-quality health information. Though this chapter is primarily dedicated to searching Google's Web search engine, many of the same tips and tricks will be applicable to other search engines.

2.2
How Do Search Engines Work?

Unlike traditional medical literature databases that are curated and populated by humans, search engines use automated computer bots to "spider" Web content, tracing as many paths through the Web as possible. These bots gather data about each Web page and return it to the search engine. The search engine then stores that data in its own database and indexes all the content to identify every possible keyword and phrase that someone might search. This means that when you search Google or another search engine, you are not searching the whole Web or the live Web – you are only searching the search engine's index. Search engines' databases have very little overlap between them, and none of them contain everything that's on the Web.

Each search engine's bots identify different data and index that data in their own way, and more importantly, each search engine will rank the results it gives you according to its own unique algorithm. Basically, you will get often completely different results depending on which search tool you use. If you aren't finding the information you want in one of them, try another tool.

Tip. In both Firefox (all versions) and Internet Explorer 7, you can search multiple search engines from the built-in search box. For more information on adding search engines to your browser, see http://mycroft.mozdev.org (Firefox users) or http://www.microsoft.com/windows/ie/searchguide/ (Internet Explorer 7 users).

Tip. If you use Firefox, add the Customize-Google extension (http://addons.mozilla.org/firefox/ 743/) to add links for searching other search engines directly into Google. This will let you compare and contrast search results in a single click. The Customize Google extension is absolutely essential for Google fanatics; in addition to adding links to competitors, you can choose to remove advertising from your search results and add many other privacy features.

Going Beyond Google

If you want to try something different than Google, hundreds of other search engines are ready and waiting for your business. There is very little overlap in coverage between the various search engines, so it's a good idea to try more than one search engine anyway. Here's a list of some of the other cool search tools out there:

Ask.com (http://www.ask.com). Ask.com is known for providing one of the best search experiences available. For many searches, Ask.com provides images, video clips, encyclopedia-type information, search suggestions for narrowing your search, and more. You can also get quick peeks at what a Web page might look like by mousing over the binoculars icon next to most results – a small snapshot of the page will pop up. Ask.com also has image, news, blog (see Chap. 15), and map searches. Ask.com's MyStuff feature lets you store your previous searches or search results, a nice feature for the researcher.

Yahoo! Search (http://search.yahoo.com). Yahoo! Search competes with Google in the sheer number of specialty search tools it offers. In addition to a general Web search engine, Yahoo! also has tools to search for audio, video, images, news, travel information, products (shopping), jobs, maps, and even a Creative Commons search to find content that you can reuse without worrying about copyright.

Live Search (http://www.live.com). Live Search is Microsoft's search tool. Live Search combines a traditional search engine with a video search tool, Microsoft HealthVault (a personalized health records system for consumers), Farecast (an airline ticket price prediction service), images, and news.

Dogpile (http://www.dogpile.com). Dogpile is a metasearch engine that combines results from all of the major search engines: Google, Ask.com, Yahoo!, and Live Search. Using Dogpile, you will only get a few results (maybe three dozen in comparison to over a million) that are the most relevant to your topic.

Country-specific search engines. Though Google, Ask.com, and some of the other search engines will generally customize their interface language and results based on your location,

(continued)

many countries have their own specialized search engines. For example, in South Korea, Naver. com is far more popular than Google. The same is true with Baidu in China. You can find search engines for your country at http://www.searchenginecolussus.com.

Specialty and alternative search engines. There are search engines out there for every interest imaginable from wine to health to green living, as well as hundreds of general search engines that want to be the next Google. If you want to find some of them, try the Alt Search Engines blog's top 100 alternative search engines lists (http://www.altsearchengines.com/category/the-top-100-lists/).

2.3
How Google Works

Many people have made careers out of trying to figure out how Google works. Because it is based on a proprietary algorithm, it's nearly impossible to say exactly how Google works, but in this section, we cover some of the basics.

2.3.1
Ranking

When ranking results, Google tries to get the most relevant results possible right at the top. To figure out which Web pages might be most relevant to you, Google performs many instantaneous calculations based on what your keywords are, what order you've placed your keywords in, how many times and where your keywords show up on a particular Web page, and most importantly, the quality of the Web site that matches your keywords.

How Google determines Web site quality is based on a number of factors, but one of the most important is the reputation of the Web site. When Google first started up, the founders had the idea to create a search engine that acted like a citation index.

A citation index is a database that focuses on the relationships created by bibliographical citations. In other words, when a journal article cites another journal article in its bibliography, a citation index records that information. With a traditional citation index like ISI Web of Science or Scopus, it's possible to see how many journal articles cited a particular article, or how many times an author's publications have been cited over time. The implication inherent in citation indices is that if an article cites another article, it is a tacit recommendation for that article.

Google's founders thought that they could use the same principles for Web sites and their links. Basically, if a Web page links to another Web page, that link is seen as a recommendation for that Web page – a marker of the linked Web site's quality. The more times a particular Web site or Web page is linked to by other Web pages, the higher it will rise in Google's rankings. This method of reputation analysis serves as the basis for PageRank, Google's algorithm.

2.3.2
What's All This?

Google has always included more than just Web pages in its search results like PDF files, Excel spreadsheets, Word documents, PowerPoint

2

presentations, and Flash movies. Since May 2007, Google's results have begun to include even more.

The Google Web search product is only one of Google's many properties on the Web. There are also Google News for news stories, Google Blog Search for searching blog posts, Google Images for finding pictures, Google Video and YouTube for finding video content, Google Local Search Results for finding local business information, Google Scholar for finding journal articles (see Chap. 6), and Google Books for searching the full contents of millions of current and out of print books. Google has begun to merge these products together in the main Web search – it's called *Universal Search*. Essentially, instead of searching three or four different Google databases to get all of the information you want, results from those other tools will show up interspersed throughout your regular Google search results.

For example, a search for don giovanni includes news results and video results from YouTube as well as regular Web results (see Fig. 1).

Wikipedia

These days, for practically every search, you'll get at least one result from Wikipedia. What is Wikipedia and why does it always show up in Google results? Wikipedia is a collaboratively written encyclopedia covering nearly every topic imaginable. It's particularly strong in technology and science fiction, but also has some coverage of medicine, science, and everything else. Wikipedia can be edited by anyone – you, your teenager, or a university professor. It's a democratizing and powerful tool, but its contents should not be taken as fact without verification. Wikipedia is an excellent starting point for most topics, however, and it ranks so highly in the Google search results because so many people link to its contents.

2.4
Basic Google Search Tips

2.4.1
Keep Your Searches Simple

As large as Google's database is, it's amazingly good at finding exactly what you need, even if you type in a single word. Don't add in a lot of extraneous words unless they are important to your search.

2.4.2
Choose Meaningful Keywords

Choosing what terms to search for is the most difficult part of searching Google. For names, places, businesses, and products, it's pretty easy to figure out what to type in the search box, but if your search has any ambiguity whatsoever, you might get stuck. Every time you search, you are trying to guess what other people think and how they express themselves. Though it's impossible to be a mind reader, try to avoid using keywords that have multiple meanings or are very generic.

2.4.3
Tailor Your Search Terms to Your Audience

If you are looking for consumer health materials to give to a patient, search for health information using consumer health terminology. For example, searching for stroke will produce more consumer-oriented Web sites while a search for cerebrovascular accident produces more results geared toward health professionals. The same is true for drug names – the generic form is more likely to find health professional-oriented information than the brand name. Nearly every profession, culture, and age group uses its own specialized terminology, and searching using that terminology will produce significantly different results.

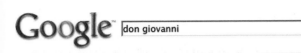 don giovanni | Search | Advanced Search / Preferences

Web   Books   Video   News

Don Giovanni - Wikipedia, the free encyclopedia - Apr 28
Don Giovanni (K.527; complete title: Il dissoluto punito, ossia il **Don Giovanni**, literally "The
Rake Punish'd, or **Don Giovanni**") is an opera in two acts ...
en.wikipedia.org/wiki/**Don_Giovanni** - 65k - Cached - Similar pages - Note this

Bistro **Don Giovanni**, Napa Valley
Bistro **Don Giovanni**, the best italian cuisine in the napa valley. Beautiful restaurant with a
rustic warm italian ambience located in the heart of the Napa ...
www.bistro**dongiovanni**.com/ - 12k - Cached - Similar pages - Note this

 Final scene of **Don Giovanni** from Amadeus
the upgraded copy here: http://www.youtube.com/watch?v ...
4 min 4 sec - ☆☆☆☆☆
www.youtube.com/watch?v=H3nqiKzB5fs

News results for **don giovanni**
 Glover-Paulus team creates a superb '**Don Giovanni**' for Chicago ... - May 2, 2008
BY ANDREW PATNER Chicago Opera Theater has scored another triumph with its new
production of "**Don Giovanni**," the last of the Mozart/Da Ponte trilogy to be ...
Chicago Sun-Times - 3 related articles »

 Don Giovanni ,"commendatore scene"
Don Giovanni:dir:John Eliot Gardiner.(the english baroque ...
6 min - ☆☆☆☆☆
www.youtube.com/watch?v=IptAkeiLzwU

Fig. 1 Google searches incorporate results from many Google products. Here, results from Google News and
YouTube (video search) are integrated into traditional Web search results

2.4.4
Add More Words to Narrow
Your Search Results

Generally, the more keywords you search for, the fewer, more specific your results will be. When adding words, stick with meaningful words. Avoid question-style searches (How many days does it take to get to the moon?).

2.4.5
All of Your Words Count

Google assumes that you want search results that include each and every one of your search terms. That means that you never have to worry about putting an AND between your search terms.

If you forget and type an AND in, Google treats it like part of your query. For example, a search for black and tan will produce different results than a search for black tan. Keep the AND in your search if it is part of a phrase – otherwise, leave it out.

2.4.6
Use Quotation Marks to Force Google to Search
for Your Terms as a Phrase

Phrase searching is one of the best and fastest ways to narrow your results. Any multiword term, name, or partial quote is a good candidate for phrase searching. By putting keywords in quotation marks, you are making Google look for your search terms exactly as you typed them – in the same order and with the same spelling. For example, a search for "journal of cardiology" will produce fewer results than searching for journal of cardiology without the quotation marks.

2.4.7
Capitalization Doesn't Matter

Google doesn't care whether you type FrEeDoM or Freedom or freedom – each is searched exactly the same.

2.4.8
Take Advantage of the Spell Check

If you mistype a word, Google will usually suggest the correct spelling for you. Simply click on the correct spelling to redo your search. Not sure how to spell a word? Give it your best shot and let Google correct you (Fig. 2).

2.4.9
Feel Lucky?

The I'm Feeling Lucky button can be a time saver. Clicking on I'm Feeling Lucky instead of hitting the Enter key or clicking on Google Search will jump you straight to the first result Google would have pulled up – you can bypass the search results page entirely. Of course, to take advantage of the I'm Feeling Lucky button, you have to be feeling a little lucky. This works best for searches for companies or anything with an official Web site.

2.4.10
Check Out the Cached Link Below Each Search Result

The cached link takes you to Google's copy of that particular Web page. Why is this a good thing? There are two major reasons: one, if the Web site is down or the page you want was moved or removed, you can still access the content through the cache; and two, the cached version will have all of your search terms highlighted, so it is easy to find exactly where your search terms are mentioned in the page, even if it is long (Fig. 3).

2.4.11
View It as HTML

Perhaps the biggest time saver of all is to use the View as HTML link shown for most PDF, Word,

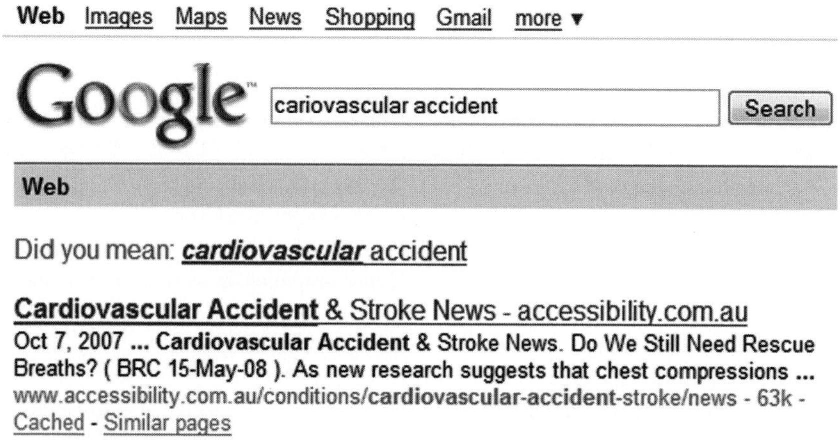

Web Images Maps News Shopping Gmail more ▼

Google [cariovascular accident] [Search]

Web

Did you mean: *cardiovascular* accident

Cardiovascular Accident & Stroke News - accessibility.com.au
Oct 7, 2007 ... **Cardiovascular Accident** & Stroke News. Do We Still Need Rescue Breaths? (BRC 15-May-08). As new research suggests that chest compressions ...
www.accessibility.com.au/conditions/**cardiovascular-accident**-stroke/news - 63k -
Cached - Similar pages

Fig. 2 Google's built-in spell check will ask "Did you mean?" for many misspellings

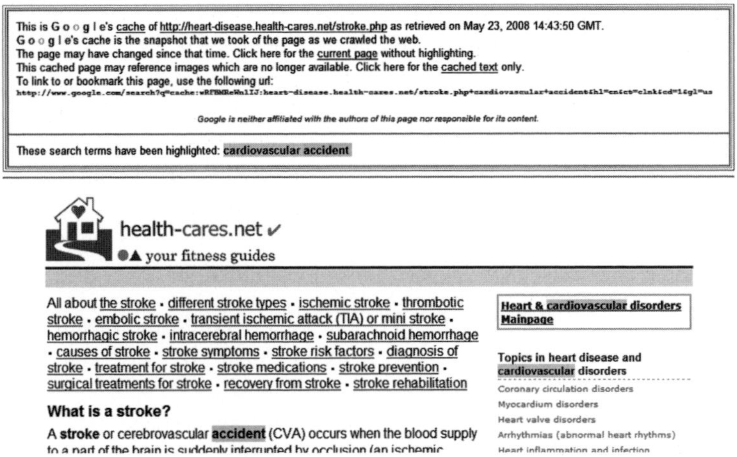

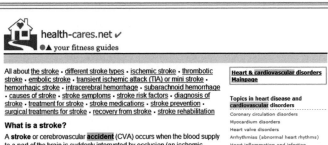

Fig. 3 Cached copies are the saved copies of Web sites in Google's database. Cached versions will have your search terms highlighted and may not include all images

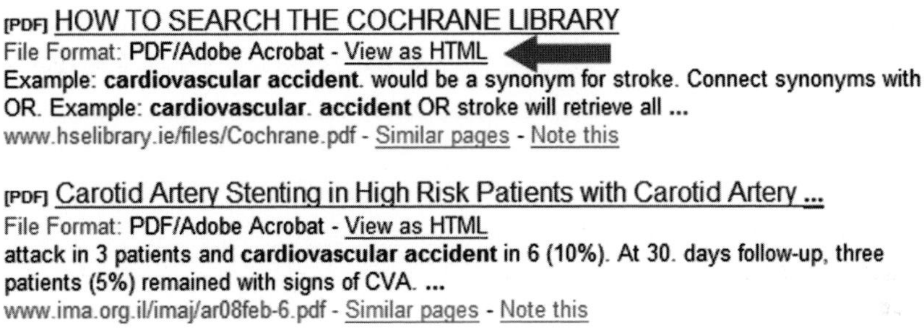

[PDF] HOW TO SEARCH THE COCHRANE LIBRARY
File Format: PDF/Adobe Acrobat - View as HTML
Example: **cardiovascular accident**. would be a synonym for stroke. Connect synonyms with
OR. Example: **cardiovascular**. **accident** OR stroke will retrieve all ...
www.hselibrary.ie/files/Cochrane.pdf - Similar pages - Note this

[PDF] Carotid Artery Stenting in High Risk Patients with Carotid Artery ...
File Format: PDF/Adobe Acrobat - View as HTML
attack in 3 patients and **cardiovascular accident** in 6 (10%). At 30. days follow-up, three
patients (5%) remained with signs of CVA. ...
www.ima.org.il/imaj/ar08feb-6.pdf - Similar pages - Note this

Fig. 4 View as HTML links show Google's Web versions of other file types (like PDF files in this example) so you don't have to open a separate program (such as Adobe Acrobat) to see content

PowerPoint, and other non-Web pages that show up in Google's results. Instead of launching a whole new program to view a search result (often only to have it be not quite what you are looking for), the View as HTML link will show you all the text from the file in Web page format (Fig. 4).

Google Advanced 3

Core Messages

› Using special search tips and tricks, you can use Google like a calculator, check for flight status information, and much more.
› Google's Advanced Search screen helps focus searches without needing to remember special search tips and commands.
› Google fanatics and power searchers can use special commands to search in extremely complex ways.
› Google's Language Tools help translate Web pages and text.

3.1
Special Tips and Tricks

For those times when you need to ramp up your Google searching technique, there are dozens of special tips and tricks you can use. Some of these tricks help refine your search, others help you broaden it, and many others open up some of Google's special built-in features beyond just search.

3.1.1
+

As a way to help you find what you are looking for without having to think of every possible spelling variation (plural forms vs. singular, for example, or conjugated verbs), Google will automatically search for term variants in most cases. What happens if you only want Web pages where a term is spelled exactly like you typed it? You have to add the plus sign (+) operator to your keyword.

Example:
+infection +control

3.1.2
−

Whereas the plus sign (+) operator adds a term to your search, the minus sign (−) operator removes a term from your search. Removing search terms has to be used with some caution, but when you need it, it's very helpful. When is it useful? The minus sign operator is primarily useful when your search results are dominated by irrelevant results or when filtering results would be beneficial. This is particularly helpful when you are searching for a person or thing whose name isn't unique.

M. Rethlefsen et al., *Internet Cool Tools for Physicians*
© Springer-Verlag Berlin Heidelberg 2009

Examples:

"delirium tremens" −beer

"Julia Roberts" −film −actress −movie

"lung cancer etiology" −tobacco

3.1.3
OR or |

In every language, there is usually more than one way to say what you mean. Searching for each individual option separately is time consuming and duplicative. Using the Boolean OR operator means you can search for more than one variant at a time.

Here's how it works. Let's say that you have a fondness for cats and dogs. When you do a typical Google search for cats dogs, you get all the pages in Google's database that talk about both cats and dogs – i.e., Google's default way to search. But looking at Fig. 1, you can see that Google is only displaying a small fraction of the material that's out there on cats and dogs. To see all the information represented by both circles, do a search for cats OR dogs. That way, the pages about both cats and dogs come up, but so do the pages on just cats and on just dogs. Using the OR operator broadens your search.

> Make sure that you capitalize the OR operator – it's the only time capitalization matters when searching Google.

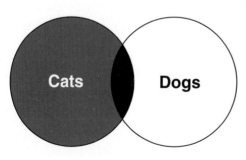

Fig. 1 Venn diagram of cats and dogs

Tip. Looking for a shortcut? The pipe symbol (|) does the same thing as the OR operator. Cats dogs is the same as cats OR dogs.

Examples:

hypertension OR "high blood pressure"

stroke OR "cerebrovascular accident"

"haemophilia b" OR "Christmas disease" OR
   "hemophilia b"

3.1.4
~

The tilde (~) is what Google calls the "fuzzy operator." Attaching the tilde (~) to any search term prompts Google to search not only for your term, but also any additional terms that Google thinks are relevant. Using the fuzzy operator can produce mixed results but is also a very powerful search tool. Instead of having to think of every possible way to express a concept, you can let Google do that work for you.

A search for ~hypertension cues Google to search for hypertension and high blood pressure, as well as the less relevant terms obesity and hypotension. A search for ~mammogram picks up mammogram, mammograms, and mammography. Where the real strength lies is with searching for less concrete concepts, such as data (~data finds data, statistics, tips, and many other relevant terms).

Example:

~mammogram ~data

> The fuzzy operator only works on single words – not on phrases. If you want to search for variants of a phrase, you'll have to do it by hand with the OR operator.

3.1.5
Calculations

Sure, you knew that Google was great at finding information, but did you know that Google can also do math? Google has a built-in calculator that can do all of the math basics for you, including addition, subtraction, multiplication, and division. If you are into fancier math, Google can help you there, too. It's capable of trigonometric functions (sin, cos, etc.), logarithms, factorials, exponentiations, and more. To use the calculator, just type your math formula into the search box (Fig. 2).

The secret to doing a conversion is using the word "in" (Fig. 3).

Examples:
150 pounds in stone
34 grams in micrograms
270 dollars in yen
500 euros in canadian dollars

Use the currency converter only as a rough guide. The rates are not updated in real time.

3.1.6
Conversions

The calculator doesn't just calculate numbers; it also calculates measure and currency conversions.

3.1.7
Phonebook

The Google PhoneBook contains residential addresses and phone numbers for the United States.

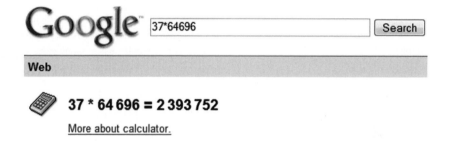

Fig. 2 Google calculator tool

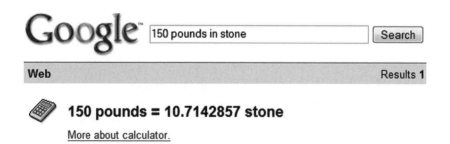

Fig. 3 Google calculator also performs measure and currency conversions

3

To use the PhoneBook, you can just type a name, city, and state or to force a residential phonebook search, use the special code phonebook: before the name, city, and state information. You'll get a phone number, address, and link to a Google Map for each result.

Example:
phonebook:nelson chicago il

Try typing a phone number in the regular search box. If it can identify the phone number, you'll often get a phonebook listing. If it can't, you may find out whose number it is by looking through the regular search results.

> Don't want your address and phone number in Google? Look yourself up, and follow the link at the bottom of the results page to remove your listing.

3.1.8
Bphonebook

Along with residential phone numbers and addresses, Google PhoneBook also contains business information. To search for phone numbers or addresses of a particular type of business, simply search for the type of business together with a location. This Google feature is notoriously unreliable, so it may not work every time you try it.

Example:
bphonebook:jewelers chicago il

3.1.9
Number Ranges

One of Google's lesser known search tools is the number range feature. Let's say that you want to purchase a stethoscope for the best deal you can. You can specify a price range by using the numbers range feature. Choose your range and put three dots between the low and high prices.

Example:
stethoscope 50…100

You can also try this trick to identify recent information by tricking Google into searching for a date range.

Example:
breast cancer 2007…2009

3.1.10
Weather

To find weather information quickly and easily, search for weather:city state. You can also find international weather with a city and country name (Fig. 4).

> Any city's weather results can be turned into a Google Gadget for your iGoogle page (see Sect. 12.3). Click on the Add to iGoogle link to add the gadget to your iGoogle page.

If you use a version of Google in a language other than English, try this special search in your language. For example, using Google.de, you can search for wetter:mannheim deutschland (Fig. 5).

3.1.11
Movie

Google's movie search makes finding movie theaters, show times, and movie ratings and reviews easy. Search for movie:city state or movie:zip code to access a handy listing of movie theaters, show times, and reviews for the area of your choice.

Example:
movie:los angeles ca

3.1.12
Flight Information

Most of the major search engines boast of some kind of flight tracking tool, and Google is no exception. To find out if a flight is on time, search for the airline code and flight number. Google will do the rest (Fig. 6).

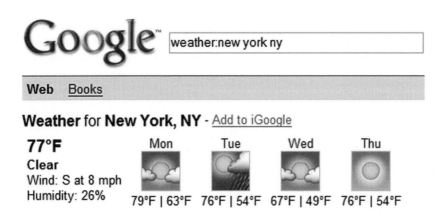

Fig. 4 Searching using the weather code gives you a 5-day forecast for the city you designate

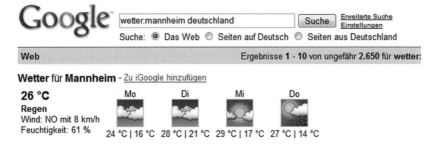

Fig. 5 Google's weather search code works internationally. This example is from Google.de

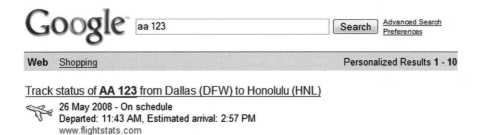

Fig. 6 Google's flight tracker tool will tell you if your flight is on time

3.1.13
Define

Google offers a couple of tricks for finding definitions. For any search, any keyword that shows up in Answers.com's dictionary will be underlined and linked to that definition in the blue bar at the top of the search results.

Better yet, though, is the special define: tool. Add define: to any word, and Google will pull together a handy list of definitions from across the Web. You can use the define: tool with slang terms; medical, technical, and scientific words; and general words.

Examples:

define:tachycardia

define:immunofluorescence

define:w00t

If the word you entered has multiple forms or variants, Google will often link to definition pages for these variants. For example, a definition search for tachycardia suggests ventricular tachycardia, superventricular tachycardia, and other forms of tachycardia.

> Want to see what changes Google is testing out for its search engine? Try SearchMash (http://www.searchmash.com) to explore Google's test site or join an experimental project (http://www.google.com/experimental/).

3.2
The Advanced Search

Chances are even if you search Google every day, you have never used the Advanced Search page. You may not even have noticed it. The Advanced Search page is linked from the main Google Web Search page to the right of the search box. You can also access it from any page of search results at the top of the screen.

Advanced Search offers many special searching tools, some of which are only accessible from the Advanced Search screen (Fig. 7):

1. The same as a regular Google search – all words entered in this box will have to be present in each search result.
2. The same as putting quotation marks around a phrase.
3. Like using the Boolean OR operator between your terms, except it doesn't work well with phrases.
4. The same as adding a minus sign to a keyword – that keyword will be removed from the search results.
5. Language limit to restrict search results to content in a single language.
6. File type restriction to limit results to content in Word documents, Excel spreadsheets, PDF files, PowerPoint presentations, or other types of content. This enables specialized searching – for example, to find presentations from a recent conference, limit to PowerPoint

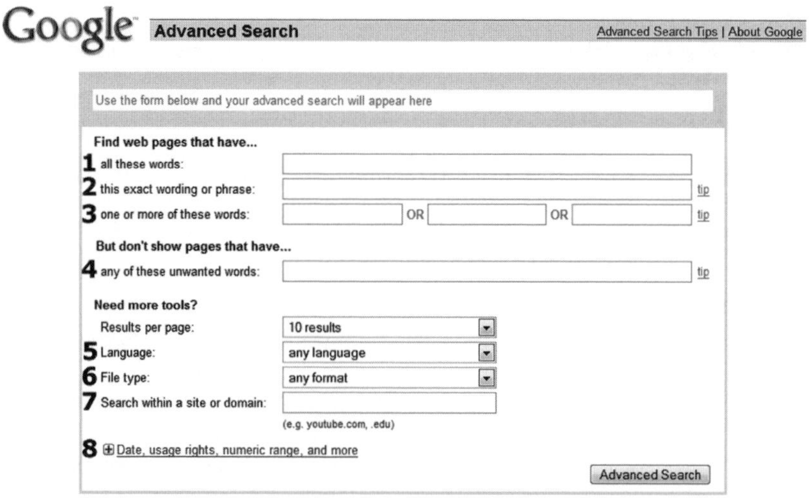

Fig. 7 Google's Advanced Search screen. Features are explained by number in Sect. 3.2

presentations. To find large reports or patient handouts, limit to PDF files.

7. Limit results to content from a specific Web site (http://www.nhs.uk) or a specific domain (e.g., .com or .gov). Limiting to a particular Web site is useful for searching sites without their own built-in search functionality. Limiting to a particular domain helps tailor the type of content Google will pull up. A domain can be a country code (.de), a domain (.com for commercial Web sites), or a combination of country code and domain (.org. uk). Sites with .org, .edu, and .gov domains tend to be considered the most reliable (.gov is for government sites, .org is for nonprofit organizations, and .edu sites are only for those sites affiliated with an institution of higher education).

8. Expand the plus box to find more search restrictions: numeric ranges, date of last update, and more.

3.3
Search Like a Pro

With the Advanced Search page and the special tips and tricks, you can do more with Google than you may have thought possible. But Google has even more search commands you can use. You can create extremely complex searches using basic Boolean logic in tandem with these search commands. Be creative!

3.3.1
Inurl

The inurl: command searches for a word in the URL (uniform resource locator) or Web address. For example, to search for information on http://www.mayo.edu, http://www.mayoclinic.com, and http://www.mayoclinic.org all at one time, you can add inurl:mayo to your search. This will pull

up any other Web pages with "mayo" in the Web address as well as the three mentioned, however.

3.3.2
Filetype

The filetype: command searches for results with a specific file format. To search for PDF files, for instance, you can add filetype:pdf to your search. Other potential file formats to limit to include PowerPoint (filetype:ppt), Flash movies (filetype:swf), Word documents (filetype:doc), or Excel spreadsheets (filetype:xls). Google indexes dozens of file types, so these are only a few examples.

3.3.3
Intitle

Most Web pages and documents have a title assigned to them by the author. Generally, the title field is the most descriptive part of any Web page, because that's what you see first in any search engine – the authors have merely a few words to peak your interest. Therefore, searching by keywords in the title field is a good way to get your results really specific. To search for good Web pages on hepatitis, you could search for intitle:hepatitis and get far fewer, yet generally more specific results.

3.3.4
Allintitle

Allintitle: is similar to intitle: except that all keywords you search for must be included in the title, not just the one attached to the special command. Searching for intitle:hepatitis treatment will get you results with the word hepatitis in the page title, but the word treatment anywhere in the page. Searching for allintitle:hepatitis treatment will ensure that both words, hepatitis and treatment, are in the page title.

3.3.5
Site

The site: command is one of the most useful tools in Google. Using the site: command allows you to limit your search results to a particular Web site (http://www.cdc.gov or http://www.nhs.uk) or a particular domain (.edu, .gov, .de). Add site:cdc.gov to search the http://www.cdc.gov site or site:uk to search only Web sites from the United Kingdom. Search within multiple sites or domains using an OR between each site.

Example:
meningitis treatment site:org OR site:edu OR
    site:cdc.gov

3.3.6
Cache

As mentioned in Sect. 2.4.10, Google stores copies of all the Web pages it indexes, and you can use these copies to find the content of Web pages that may have disappeared from the live Internet. In addition to the Cached link present for most Google pages, it's possible to search for a cached copy of a Web page directly using the cache: command. For example, try cache:http://www.medlineplus.gov.

The cache: command won't always retrieve the Web page you need. Another place to try to locate old Web content is the Internet Archive's Wayback Machine (http://www.archive.org/). The Wayback Machine stores copies of Web sites over time, and though it is not 100% comprehensive, it contains an enormous amount of Web content.

3.4
Language Tools

One of Google's most impressive offerings is Language Tools (http://www.google.com/language_tools). Language tools feature translation capabilities as well as another place to change the Google interface language or to search Google in a local domain (e.g., http://www.google.de). One recent feature added to the Language Tools Web page is search translation. Type a word in your language, pick the language to translate it into, and Google will search for the translated version.

Google can translate words, chunks of text, and entire Web pages almost instantaneously. To translate a Web page, simply enter the Web address of the page you want to translate into the box and select the appropriate language for translation. For accessing only the text and Web page translation tools, an alternate site is http://translate.google.com/.

Along with the major European languages, Google's Language Tools can also translate Chinese, Japanese, Arabic, Russian, and more. More languages are added frequently.

Make use of the translation features built into the Google Toolbar for extra translation power. Another handy Google translation tool is the gTranslate Firefox extension that translates any selected word or piece of text as a right-click option (https://addons.mozilla.org/en-US/firefox/addon/918).

If you are a Google Talk (or Gmail with built-in Google Talk) instant messaging user, you can chat with Google's translation bots to get real-time translation via instant messaging. See http://googletalk.blogspot.com/2007/12/merry-christmas-god-jul-and.html for more information.

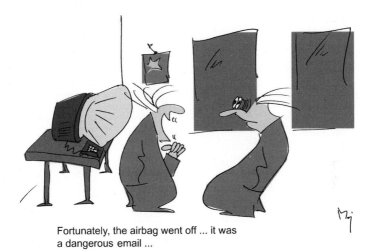

Fortunately, the airbag went off ... it was
a dangerous email ...

Google Health

4

Core Messages

> Google has a strong healthcare focus.
> Google Co-op provides searchers with refinements on healthcare-related searches that direct users to curated, high-quality health resources.
> The new Google Health product is a personal health record system for consumers.

4.1
Finding Health Information on Google

Consumers and medical professionals alike use Google to find health information. Studies have shown that 80% of Americans have used a search engine to find health information for themselves or family members.

Google knows this and takes their role in providing consumer health and medical information very seriously. They want to provide the best health information possible, particularly to consumers. One of the first initiatives Google took was a rather convoluted tool called *Google Co-op*. Google Co-op was created to allow health organizations and health professionals to select high-quality consumer health and medical information out on the Web and share those sites with others in Google.

When anyone does a search on Google for most health conditions, diseases, symptoms, or drug names, a number of refinements will pop up at the top of the page. Refinements will vary by topic, but generally include the options "For health professionals" and "For patients." Other refinements may include "Tests/diagnosis," "Symptoms," "Side effects," "Clinical trials," or "Alternative therapy." Clicking on one of these refinements will trigger Google to display results with the hand-selected, labeled results on top. Each result displays the selected label plus who labeled that result.

Google worked with several major United States healthcare organizations like the Mayo Clinic, the National Library of Medicine, the Health on the Net Foundation, and the Centers for Disease Control and Prevention to produce the original listings of these special health results, but anyone can create a Google Co-op account and label health information on their own. At least one physician, Enoch Choi, has done so, and now you can see the health Web sites he likes labeled along with those labeled by WebMD and others (Figs. 1 and 2).

4

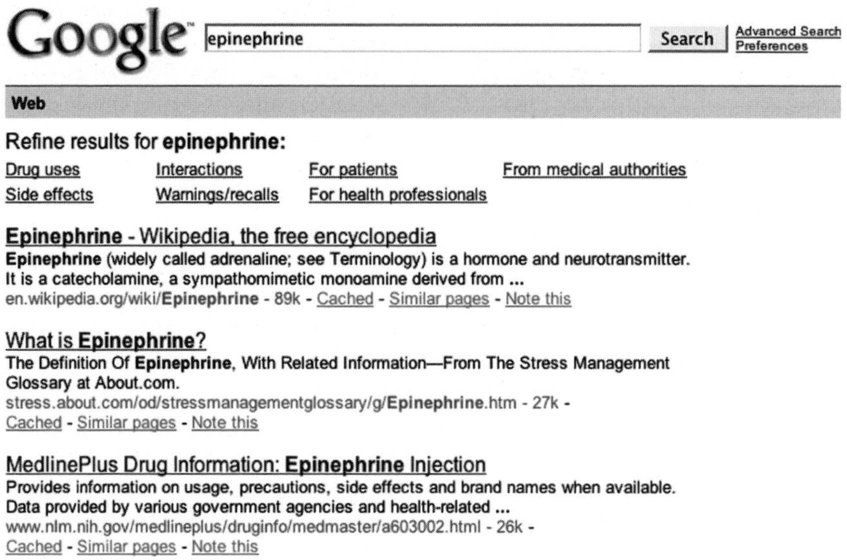

Google™ | epinephrine | Search | Advanced Search
                                                                      Preferences

Web

Refine results for epinephrine:

Drug uses   Interactions   For patients   From medical authorities
Side effects   Warnings/recalls   For health professionals

Epinephrine - Wikipedia, the free encyclopedia
Epinephrine (widely called adrenaline; see Terminology) is a hormone and neurotransmitter.
It is a catecholamine, a sympathomimetic monoamine derived from ...
en.wikipedia.org/wiki/**Epinephrine** - 89k - Cached - Similar pages - Note this

What is **Epinephrine**?
The Definition Of **Epinephrine**, With Related Information—From The Stress Management
Glossary at About.com.
stress.about.com/od/stressmanagementglossary/g/**Epinephrine**.htm - 27k -
Cached - Similar pages - Note this

MedlinePlus Drug Information: **Epinephrine** Injection
Provides information on usage, precautions, side effects and brand names when available.
Data provided by various government agencies and health-related ...
www.nlm.nih.gov/medlineplus/druginfo/medmaster/a603002.html - 26k -
Cached - Similar pages - Note this

Fig. 1 Health-related searches cause Google to display refinements. This search on epinephrine shows refinements to information for health professionals and several other subcategories

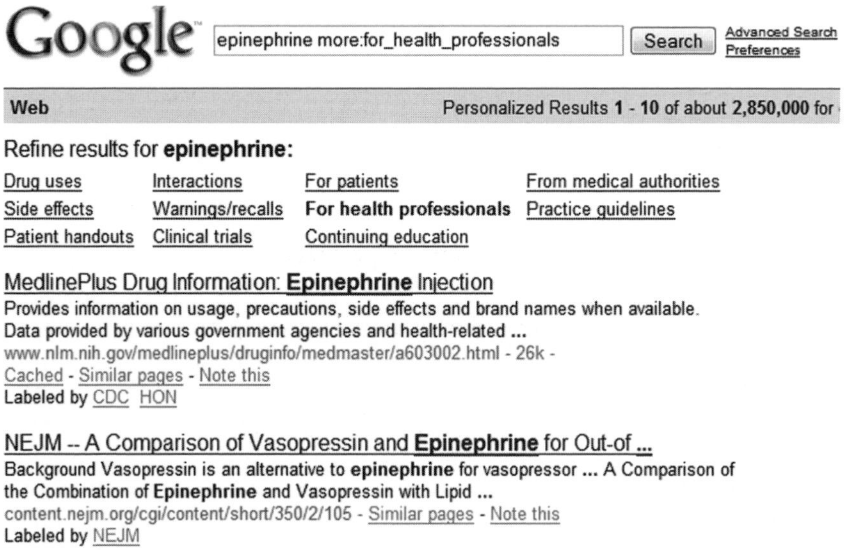

Google™ | epinephrine more:for_health_professionals | Search | Advanced Search
                                                                      Preferences

Web   Personalized Results **1 - 10** of about **2,850,000** for

Refine results for epinephrine:

Drug uses   Interactions   For patients   From medical authorities
Side effects   Warnings/recalls   **For health professionals** Practice guidelines
Patient handouts   Clinical trials   Continuing education

MedlinePlus Drug Information: **Epinephrine** Injection
Provides information on usage, precautions, side effects and brand names when available.
Data provided by various government agencies and health-related ...
www.nlm.nih.gov/medlineplus/druginfo/medmaster/a603002.html - 26k -
Cached - Similar pages - Note this
Labeled by CDC HON

NEJM -- A Comparison of Vasopressin and **Epinephrine** for Out-of ...
Background Vasopressin is an alternative to **epinephrine** for vasopressor ... A Comparison of
the Combination of **Epinephrine** and Vasopressin with Lipid ...
content.nejm.org/cgi/content/short/350/2/105 - Similar pages - Note this
Labeled by NEJM

Fig. 2 Clicking on health search refinements launches searchers into vetted content. Vetted content is labeled by the organization or individual who selected it for that particular topic and refinement

4.2
Google Health (http://www.google.com/health)

In late spring 2008, Google released Google Health. Google Health, which was created under the advisement of physicians and health-care organizations, is Google's foray into personal health records. Since a very large percentage of Google searches are about health and medicine, Google saw a need to provide reliable health information, which they began in Google Co-op. Google Health goes far beyond Google Co-op to offer patients and consumers a central-ized place to store health records, check on drug interactions, and interface with their health-care systems (Cleveland Clinic is an early partner) and pharmacies (Walgreens is another partner) (Fig. 3).

Patients can import health records from selected providers as well as enter in their own information about medications, allergies, immunizations, test results, and procedures. When medications are entered, Google Health will automatically check for and display potential drug interactions. For each condition entered, links lead to consumer health content, both text and images, provided by A.D.A.M. Additional information pulled from discussion groups (Google Groups), Google News, and related Google searches is also displayed (Figs. 4 and 5).

Consumers can also use search tools to locate physicians and other health practitioners in their area. This tool is primarily based on content already in the Google search engine, so it is not as reliable as AMA Doctor Finder or similar tools for consumers. It does, however, help patients locate physicians across the globe.

Though at the time of writing this book, Google Health is brand new and untested in wide release, it promises to be one of a number of interesting new personal health management and personal health record systems being devel-oped. Other players in this market are Revolution Health and Microsoft Health Vault.

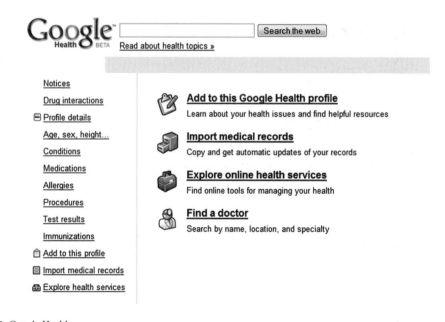

Fig. 3 Google Health

4

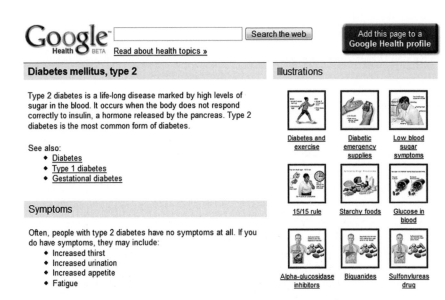

Fig. 4 Consumer health information contained in Google Health for diabetes mellitus type 2

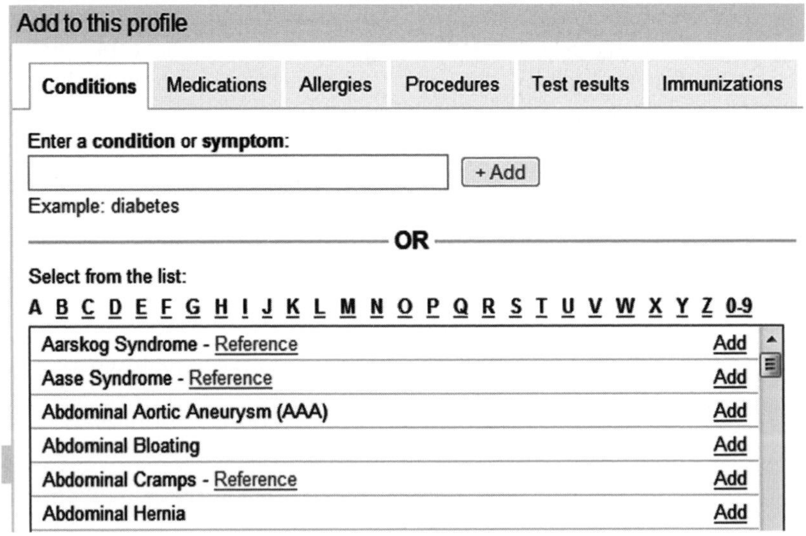

Fig. 5 Adding conditions to a health profile in Google Health

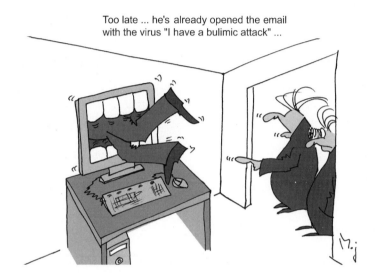

Too late ... he's already opened the email with the virus "I have a bulimic attack" ...

Personalizing Google

5

Core Messages

> Update your Google Preferences to customize the search engine's language and display.

> Google Subscribed Links let you add custom search results into Google, including drug monographs from ePocrates or other health sources.

> Refind search results and Web pages you've visited using Web History.

> Google personalizes search results for you based on your Web History.

Google is a huge search engine – how do you make it yours? There are many ways to personalize Google, both in appearance and functionality. In this section, we cover some of the basics of customizing your Google experience.

5.1
Preferences

One of the simplest ways to customize Google is to use Google's built-in Preferences. To access the Google Preferences menu, follow the link to the right of the Google search box.

By default, Google displays 10 search results per page. You can use the Preferences options to boost this to 20, 50, or even 100 results per page.

You can also use the Preferences to set the default interface language, choose SafeSearch Preferences to remove questionable content from Google's results, and more. Just click on Save Preferences when you've selected your options, and Google will put a cookie in your browser so that each time you use Google, the Preferences will remain the same. If you clear your cookies, you will need to reset your preferences.

Tip. The Google engineers have a good sense of humor. Try scrolling through the interface language options available – you might be surprised at what you find! Just be careful – if you don't know the Klingon word for English, you'll have some trouble resetting your preferences.

Another feature accessible in Preferences are Subscribed Links (also available directly at http://www.google.com/coop/sl). Subscribed Links is just what it sounds like – it invites users to subscribe to various content sources, the links for which will show up in Google search results if relevant. Google Subscribed Links is still rather experimental and has not gained a lot of momentum, but there are several health- and medicine-related Subscribed Links providers worth subscribing to, including ePocrates (Fig. 1).

To access the directory of Subscribed Links providers, click on Subscribed Links directory in

M. Rethlefsen et al., *Internet Cool Tools for Physicians*
© Springer-Verlag Berlin Heidelberg 2009

MedlinePlus Drug Information: **Epinephrine** Injection

Provides information on usage, precautions, side effects and brand names when available.
Data provided by various government agencies and health-related ...
www.nlm.nih.gov/medlineplus/druginfo/medmaster/a603002.html - 26k -
Cached - Similar pages - Note this

Epocrates Information for **epinephrine** - Manage my Subscribed Links

 For entire: Monograph
For only: Adult Dosage
For only: Adverse Reactions
online.epocrates.com

Adrenalin (**Epinephrine**) drug description - FDA approved labeling ...

Find Adrenalin (**Epinephrine**) medication description and FDA approved drug information
including side effects, interactions and patient labeling.
www.rxlist.com/cgi/generic/epi.htm - 39k - Cached - Similar pages - Note this

Fig. 1 Searching for epinephrine when ePocrates is a Subscribed Link puts ePocrates drug monograph listings directly into Google search results

Preferences (alternately, go directly to http://www.google.com/coop/subscribedlinks/directory/All_categories). Click on the Subscribe button to subscribe to a provider. Using Subscribed Links does require a Google Account and also requires logging in to the account whenever you are searching Google to access the subscriptions in your results. The main health- and medicine-related Subscribed Links providers are:

- ePocrates (http://www.google.com/coop/profile?user=012225514705487255494)
- Medscape (http://www.google.com/coop/profile?user=007637489950372872184)
- MedPage Today (http://www.google.com/coop/profile?user=010149774059323981942)
- KidsHealth (http://www.google.com/coop/profile?user=004954636874575689593)

Tip. For Delicious users (see Sect. 18.4 for information about Delicious), you can build your Delicious links into Google search results using Subscribed Links. See http://sandbox.sourcelabs.com/kibbutz/generate.php for details. This does require entering your username and password for your Delicious account on a third-party site.

5.2
Web History and Personalized Results

Google wants to make your search results personal. Even without logging into Google, Google will personalize search results based on previous searches in a single search session. For instance, if your first search was for "coffee" and your second search was for "java," Google might pull up more results about java related to coffee than the programming language or the country. But Google can get even more personal.

In theory, for every search you perform, Google can pull up results tailored to your personal needs. How does Google achieve this level of personalization? Google can personalize your search results based on your Google search history and your Web browsing history, but only if you allow it.

The two major ways Google tracks personal information about you and your Web History are through the Google Account and the Google Toolbar. Any time you sign up for a Google service or product, you create a Google Account. If you are logged into this account (e.g., a Gmail account) while you are doing Web searches, Google will track your search history for you. You can access the search history at any time from the main Google search page or the results pages.

The search history tracks not only the search terms you enter into the regular Google search engine, but also searches in the other Google search products, like Google Video, Google Images, and Google News. Any search result that you click on is also recorded so that you can easily relocate a particular Web site you may have clicked on. The search history in part is what enables Google to tailor search results.

Though the search history is useful for you and for Google, the Web History is the real powerhouse behind search personalization. The Web History feature is only available for Google Toolbar users.

The Google Toolbar is a handy extension for your Web browser. Versions are available for Firefox and Internet Explorer. With the Google Toolbar, you can perform Google searches directly from the toolbar's search box, bookmark Web sites with Google Bookmarks, check spelling, and much more (Fig. 2).

Through the Google Toolbar, Google can track every Web site that you visit. This isn't a default option, however; Google gives you plenty of warning before you make the decision to turn it on. Should you turn on this option, Google will keep a record of all the Web sites you visit by date and time and will store a copy of that Web page for you.

Enabling the Web History gives you two major benefits. First of all, you can browse or search your Web History at any time – not just the search terms, but the full contents of any Web page you had visited since you turned on the Web History. This means that you have a much better chance of refinding a Web page you visited a few months ago, even if you don't remember much about it. Secondly, the Web History will help Google personalize any future search results by figuring in the type of Web content you have looked at in the past.

If you're not sure you want Google tracking your Web History or search history, you can permanently turn off that feature in your account (http://www.google.com/history/). You can also pause your Web History temporarily on the Web History page (look for the Pause link) or erase your Web History (Fig. 3).

There are several Firefox extensions that help you customize your Google experience. Look for CustomizeGoogle (http://www.customizegoogle.com/) and GooglePreview (https://addons.mozilla.org/en-US/firefox/addon/189).

5.3
iGoogle

To get really personal with Google, you can create a personalized start page. Google calls their personalized start page product iGoogle.

Fig. 2 The Google Toolbar adds a Google search box, links to Google tools and services, and many other useful features to your Internet Explorer or Firefox browser

5

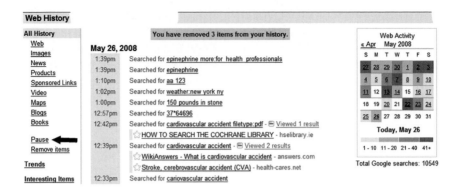

Fig. 3 Google Web History tracks your search history and what Web sites you've visited. You can pause tracking at any time from the Web History Web page

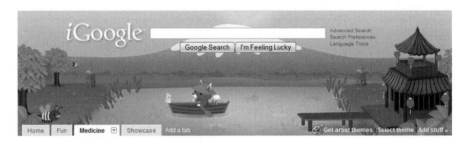

Fig. 4 One of iGoogle's many available themes

Using iGoogle, you can choose to pretty up your Google search page with a selection of different themes (http://www.google.com/ig/ directory?=en&type=themes) (Fig. 4). There's a lot more to iGoogle that we'll be covering in greater detail in Sect. 12.3.

Core Messages

> Google Scholar is Google's academically oriented search engine.

> Google Scholar contains journal articles, preprints, books, patents, and other scholarly resources.

> Google Scholar is a citation index – it lets you track what articles have been cited where, and it orders results by how often an article is cited.

> Searching Google Scholar is similar to searching the regular Google search engine, but with a few advanced search tricks as well.

arly? That's a bit of a mystery, but there are a couple of general areas Google Scholar covers:

- Journal articles
- Other scholarly databases
- Institutional repositories
- Higher education Web sites
- Patents

In medicine, Google Scholar can be hit or miss. It contains a large number of PubMed citations, but not all of them, nor are the citations particularly current. Google also worked with many of the scientific, technical, and medical print and online publishers like Elsevier (Science Direct), HighWire, Wiley (InterScience), and the Nature Publishing Group to include their journal articles.

6.1
What Is Google Scholar? (http://scholar. google.com)

You've heard of Google, but have you ever heard of Google Scholar? Chances are you haven't. Google Scholar is a Google product still under development, even though it has been around since 2003. Unlike Google, which searches as much of the Web as possible, Google Scholar restricts itself to what it considers "scholarly" Web sites. So, what does Google consider schol-

6.2
Why Should You Use Google Scholar?

A couple of things make Google Scholar unique. First of all, Google Scholar searches the full text of articles, not just the title and abstract. This means that you might find some articles you wouldn't have found using PubMed (see Chap. 8) or another article database, but it also means that you will often get a large number of results. The large number of results is not always important, though, because, first of all, Google Scholar

M. Rethlefsen et al., *Internet Cool Tools for Physicians*
© Springer-Verlag Berlin Heidelberg 2009

6

will only ever show you the first 1,000 results, even if it says there are 100,000,000 results. Most importantly, however, the results you do see are the ones that Google Scholar thinks are most relevant to your search – they are not just in reverse chronological order. This means that you can often find a great article or two on your topic right at the top of your results.

This may sound familiar – after all, Google works the same way, putting the most relevant results first. Google Scholar, like Google, determines how relevant a result is to your search based on a number of factors, one of which is how many times it was cited. In Google Scholar, you will almost always see the most heavily cited articles first. Because of this emphasis on citation, Google Scholar is excellent for finding key or classic articles on a topic.

Relevance ranking can be a detriment to physicians, though. Instead of seeing the latest research or the newest practice guidelines, you're likely to get older, potentially out of date material. You can change how the Google Scholar results sort to emphasize "recent articles" (look

for the link at the top of the results page), but you still won't find the most current articles – just more current articles than you would otherwise.

> Google Scholar is also a citation index – in fact, it's the only free citation index available. This means that by searching Google Scholar, you can figure out who cited an article. Want to see who cited your paper? Do an author search and look for the "Cited by" link underneath each citation.

6.3
Searching Google Scholar

Searching Google Scholar is as simple as searching Google. All you really need to do is type in your keywords and look through the results. As mentioned above, however, Google Scholar is a beta product – this means it can be a bit finicky, and you may not always be sure what you will get and what you are seeing (Fig. 1).

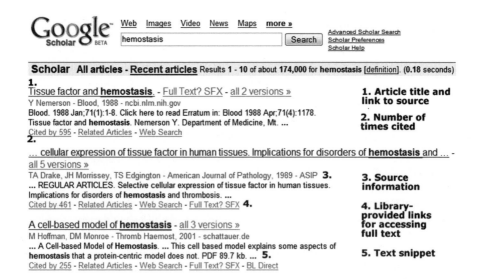

Fig. 1 Understanding Google Scholar search results. This graphic shows the major features available from Google Scholar results: links to full text, citation information, source information, library-provided links to full text, and text snippets

Because Google Scholar searches institutional repositories, educational Web sites, publishers' Web sites, and databases across the Web, the disparate sources it pulls information from may contain duplicate records for the same item. Most of the time, Google Scholar is smart enough that it can merge these together into one record with a link to the duplicates. This means that the link to the full text you see in the results may be a link to a manuscript or an archived copy of an article, and not necessarily to the article on the publisher's Web site. Many times, this is helpful, because you may be able to get access to an article you wouldn't normally be able to access – but it does leave the results a little messy.

Many citations don't link to the full text at all. This is particularly true with older citations (Google Scholar contains records to items thousands of years old as well as more current citations) and books, dissertations, and other nonarticle citations. The reason is that Google Scholar's content largely comes from mining bibliographies – this is why it has such a huge range of materials from all disciplines and time periods, and this is how it works as a citation index. Most of the time, the article citations without links to full text won't be enough to help you find the real articles – basic information like volume, issue, and page numbers is usually removed from the citation. Check with your medical librarian to help track down any elusive citations you need.

Google Scholar by default adds a "Library Search" link to book citations. Clicking on the Library Search link will take you to Open WorldCat, a tool that can help you locate books in libraries nearest you. Simply type in your Zip Code (United States) or country name (other countries). This tool is most useful for American physicians, though major libraries in most countries have their books listed in Open WorldCat.

You can search Google Scholar by subject as well as by author, source (journal name), and even date range. Try the Advanced Search page or the advanced commands to use these search methods.

Basic Search Tips

Keep your searches simple. Try to use just a few keywords that are very pertinent to your topic. You don't need to worry about using AND between your search terms – Google Scholar will automatically search for just those articles with all of your terms.

Use quotation marks to force Google Scholar to search for multiple words together as a phrase. For example, instead of searching for heart disease prevention, try searching for "heart disease" prevention. You'll get fewer results that will be more specific to your topic.

Try the advanced search page. The advanced search page, available as a link from the main Google Scholar page or the top of any results page (http://scholar.google.com/advanced_scholar_search), contains a number of very helpful tools: date limits, author searching, journal title searching, and even a way to limit your search by a general subject area.

Learn advanced search commands. Some of the advanced search commands in Google Scholar are the same as in the regular Google search engine – using quotation marks for a phrase, for example. Others are unique to Google Scholar. See the Advanced Commands box for a list of advanced search commands with examples.

Set your preferences. Before you even begin searching Google Scholar, you should set your searching preferences. In the Preferences menu, you can associate yourself with a library so that you can access the full-text articles your medical library might provide. You can also set up links to import Google Scholar citations into a bibliographic management tool, including EndNote, Reference Manager, and RefWorks. If you use Zotero (see Sect.

6

19.3.1), using the EndNote option will let you add Google Scholar citations to Zotero in one click. The preferences are available from the main Google Scholar page (look to the right of the search box) or directly at http://scholar.google.com/scholar_preferences.

Advanced Commands

author:
Search for an author by last name or by last name and initials
author:smith
author:"jd smith"

intitle:
Search for a word or phrase in an article or book title
intitle:aggression
intitle:"crash course"

allintitle:
Search for all search terms in an article or book title

allintitle: "video games" aggression adolescents −
Remove a word from your search
"video games" −violence flowers −author: flowers
+
Add a word to your search exactly as typed
+violence +teenagers

site:
Search for materials from a particular Web site
site:nejm.org "chest tube" ...
Search for items in a specific date range
sea-blue histiocytosis 1999...2009

OR
Search for items with either of your terms
"heart attack" OR "myocardial infarction"
red OR green apples

Putting It Together
site:nejm.org author:pitt "heart attack" OR "myocardial infarction" −protocol 2000...2008

You are coughing too much ...
Now closing all windows ...

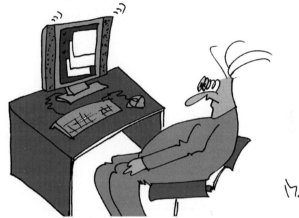

Core Messages

> People search engines can help you locate elusive phone numbers, addresses, and email addresses.

> Find email addresses and other contact information for professional colleagues using PubMed.

7.1
People Search

Finding people on the Web is notoriously difficult. Unless the person you are trying to track down has an uncommon name, a large or well-established Web presence, or is a celebrity, chances are you may have trouble finding them using a traditional search engine like Google. The tips in Chaps. 2 and 3 like the phonebook search (see Sect. 3.1.7) and using quotation marks around names (see Sect. 2.4.6) will help, but even then, you are still restricted to the content that Google searches. A lot of person-specific information is hidden in databases and behind firewalls, meaning even with the best Google searching techniques, it's still difficult

to find everything. In this chapter, we'll cover a few databases and tips that can help you track down people and their email addresses.

7.1.1
Phone Directories

Often, the easiest way to track down someone is by using a phonebook. In Sect. 3.1.7, we covered using Google to search for United States phone numbers and addresses, but there are online phonebooks for most countries. A good listing is available at http://www.numberway.com/.

7.1.2
People Search Engines

There are numerous search engines out there devoted solely to finding people. Here are some you might want to try:

- **Spock (http://www.spock.com).** Spock searches Web results and has its own international people database. You can search by name, location, or keyword – or a combination.
- **ZabaSearch (http://www.zabasearch. com).** ZabaSearch is a scarily good tool for tracking down people in the United States. It

M. Rethlefsen et al., *Internet Cool Tools for Physicians*
© Springer-Verlag Berlin Heidelberg 2009

includes phone numbers and addresses pulled from public records. You can search by name, phone number, or social security number. The only trick to using ZabaSearch is trying to sort the current, good information from the outdated information – both are included.

- **Spokeo (http://www.spokeo.com).** Spokeo searches for people in social networks (see Chap. 20 for information about social networks) and anywhere else people have profiles, like Flickr. You can enter in someone's email address and find out which services they have accounts on in a matter of seconds. It's primarily designed as an aggregator of social network content, meaning instead of logging on to the 41 different services and tracking down your friends on each place, Spokeo will let you access them all in one place.

- **Pipl (http://www.pipl.com).** Pipl is an international people search engine with amazingly good results. It searches international phone books, many institutional directories, and other content not accessible in regular search engines, as well as offers links to paid services for tracking down even more information.

- **Infobel (http://www.infobel.be).** Infobel provides a directory of international people search tools, primarily phone books.

- **Yahoo! People Search (http://people. yahoo.com).** Yahoo! People Search is perhaps the most popular and well used of all people search engines. It offers a reverse phone directory and email search tool, though the phone directory information is United States specific.

- **Wink (http://www.wink.com).** Another people search tool.

- **PeekYou (http://www.peekyou.com).** PeekYou can help you find people's usernames for various services as well as basic information like location.

7.1.3
Medical Directories

Finding physicians online is made easier through Google Health (http://www.google.com/health, see Sect. 4.2), but there are also physician directories available from professional societies.

AMA Doctor Finder (http://webapps.ama-assn.org/doctorfinder/home.html) is a comprehensive directory of physicians in the United States, even if they are not members of the American Medical Association. The information in AMA Doctor Finder includes (for most physicians) licensure information, medical school and residency programs, and contact information.

Finding certification information is made available through the American Board of Medical Specialties "Is Your Doctor Certified?" tool (http://www.abms.org/newsearch.asp). Registration is required to use this service. If neither of these tools is productive, many specialties have their own databases of providers. A good list of these databases is available through MEDLINEplus (http://www.nlm.nih.gov/medlineplus/directories.html).

7.2
Email

Email, short for electronic mail, is one of the most used services on the Internet. It allows delivering text and documents to your destination nearly always within minutes of being sent. That's great if the email address of your destination is known. However, what can you do if you don't know it or the one you have is not working? In this section, you will learn the most important techniques on how you can find those elusive email addresses.

The email address lets your computer know how to get the email to the right person. To be able to find someone's address, you need to understand how email addresses are composed. Each email address is a string of the form jmiller@example.com. It should be read as "jmiller at example dot com." It is written with no spaces whatsoever and consists of the following established parts (Fig. 1):

- Local part of the address, usually the user-name of the recipient
- @ (the "at" symbol), which separates the local part from the domain part of the address
- Domain part of the address, which may be a host name or domain name

Domain names are unique identifiers for the organization that manages the email accounts. Some examples are:

- hotmail.com – Windows Live Hotmail Internet access provider
- aol.com – AOL Internet access provider
- whitehouse.gov – United States White House
- mayo.edu – Mayo Clinic
- chisuk.org.uk – Complementary Healthcare Information Service – UK

Tip. In case you have an email address that's not working, you should first verify whether it's misspelled, and check that the entire address is written with no spaces. Misspellings in the recipient's name or well-known domain names are easily identifiable.

7.3 Finding Email Addresses

Finding the right email address for the person you want to contact might be time consuming since there is no complete phone directory of people's or organizations' email addresses. Another problem is that, due to spamming, many email addresses have been removed from Web pages.

7.3.1 Previous Messages

Use the search function in your email to locate addresses for people you may have sent or received email from previously. If you find an email, use the address in the line "From:" or "To:" ignoring angle brackets "< >" or parentheses "( )," which might frame the address, e.g., use jmiller@example.com instead of <jmiller@example.com>. If only a name is visible, double click it, and generally a new window will disclose the email address.

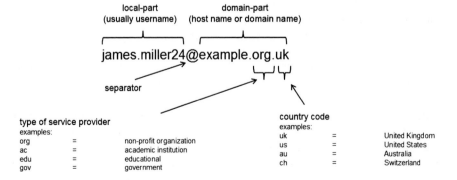

Fig. 1 The anatomy of an email address

7

7.3.2
Email Directories

There are many directories of email addresses; however, they are all limited in scope. Many find email addresses by snooping around Web pages, by watching newsgroups, and through direct submission by individuals or organizations. Some of them charge a fee for lookups.

This is a small selection of Web directories useful when looking for an email address:

- **Yahoo! People Search (http://people. yahoo.com).** As mentioned in Sect. 7.1, Yahoo! People Search allows you to search for email addresses.
- **My Email Address Is (http://my.email. address.is).** My Email Address Is is a meta-search engine returning results from Yahoo!, Switchboard, InfoSpace, and Look4U.
- **FreshAddress (http://freshaddress.com/ stayintouch.cfm).** FreshAddress is a free worldwide registry of old and current email addresses. Old addresses can be registered along with the new one. Therefore, if the email address you have for someone is not working anymore, you might be able to find the new one in case the change has been submitted. Registration is required to use FreshAddress.

In case it is unlikely that the person you are looking is named on a Web site or uses newsgroups or other Internet services, don't spend too much time here. Unfortunately, still only a minority of people registers their own email address with one of these services.

7.3.3
Ph and LDAP Phonebooks

If the person whose address you are looking for works in a large organization, you might consider consulting Ph and LDAP online phonebooks. These two tools are commonly used by larger organizations, particularly universities, to keep their internal phonebooks online. A good site listing public Ph and LDAP online directories is eMailman (http://www.emailman.com).

7.3.4
PubMed

If the person you want to contact has published scientific articles (or if you suspect they may have), perform an author search in PubMed (http://www.pubmed.gov). In the Limits tab, enter your quarry's name in the Search by Author field (see Sect. 8.3.2 for more information on using the PubMed Limits tab). Click on the authors' names listed in the PubMed results to get to the Abstract view for each result. If an email address was entered into the PubMed database, it will be listed.

Email addresses are supplied by more and more journals, but not all of them, and those that do provide them generally list them for only the corresponding author. If the email address is not listed in PubMed, however, try looking at the full-text article, as many times the full articles list email addresses for more than just the corresponding author. (For more about accessing full-text articles, see Sect. 8.5 about accessing articles via PubMed and Chap. 6 about Google Scholar.)

7.3.5
Search the Web

When in doubt, search the Web. Remember that Google is not the only search engine out there. For a truly comprehensive search, try at least the four major search engines: Google (http://www.google. com), Ask (http://www.ask.com), Yahoo! (http:// search.yahoo.com), and MSN or Live Search (http://www.live.com). If it's likely that the person has published scientific articles, add Google Scholar (http://scholar.google.com) to that list.

Usually, typing only the given name and family name will return many useless hits when looking for an email address. Why? First, unless the name is very rare, you'll get results for many different people all together, so it may be difficult to differentiate between them. Second, only a small percentage of results will contain an email address. How can you improve your search? If you are looking for the email address of a person with a rare name, e.g., Rosemary Montabaur, try the following strategies:

- rosemary montabaur email
- rosemary montabaur at

If the family name is very rare, e.g., Paperin, you may try omitting the given name since it might not show up in the email address:

- paperin email
- paperin at

What should you consider if the name is common, such as James Miller? Try to reduce the number of hits by adding as much information as you have about the person, including the name of city where the person is living or working, the person's job title or company, or any other personal details:

- james miller email boston
- james miller at boston

7.3.6
Find the Domain First

If you know the domain part of the person's email address already, things get easier. Before you spend a lot of time searching for someone on the Web, you might invest some time looking for the domain name before you start. If you know the organization the person is working with, try to find its Web site. It's likely that any email address on the organizational Web site will have the same domain as the individual's.

If the person works at an institution publishing scientific articles, try finding the organization's domain in PubMed. Let's say John Miller is work-

ing at the University of Appenzell. Select the Tag Term affiliation in PubMed's Limits tab and perform a search with the terms university appenzell. This retrieves all citations where an author lists an affiliation with the University of Appenzell. Choose any article in the results to find the domain uniappenzell.ch. Knowing this domain, search in a regular search engine with a strategy such as:

- john miller uniappenzell.ch
- jmiller uniappenzell.ch
- john.miller@uniappenzell.ch
- john_miller@uniappenzell.ch
- miller@uniappenzell.ch (this will also return addresses with strings in front of "miller")

Finding common names in large organizations might be impossible, however, since it's likely that they run out of simple email names. Many times, for common names, numbers get appended to the address, e.g., john.miller17@uniappenzell.ch or jmiller45@uniappenzell.ch.

7.3.7
University Directories

Many universities provide faculty directories on their Web sites. If your correspondent works at a university, for example, the London Business School of the University of London, first locate the university Web site. You may need to search or browse through the university's Web site to locate the directory. Some may be restricted to faculty, staff, and student use.

7.3.8
Professional Associations

Is the person whose email address you are looking for member of a professional association? If so, you might be able to get their email address through the association. However, most online directories of professional associations are restricted to their members. If you are not a member, you might ask a member you know for help.

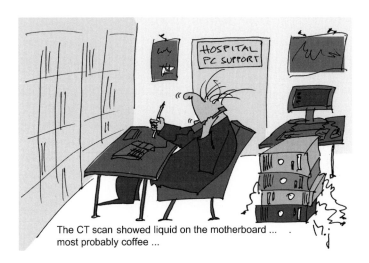

The CT scan showed liquid on the motherboard ... . most probably coffee ...

PubMed

Core Messages

> PubMed is the premiere database for searching the biomedical literature.

> PubMed offers many options to refine searches, save searches and selected citations, and retrieve full-text articles.

> Finding full-text articles may require pay per view from publishers, setting up a document delivery account, or finding free content from publishers and authors.

8.1
PubMed (http://www.pubmed.gov)

PubMed is designed to make searching for medical literature easy. Instead of having to worry about finding the right terms, PubMed does the thinking for you – it interprets the words you type into the search box and tries to match those words with the medical subject headings, author names, journal titles, and other terms it thinks that you mean. And, there is the problem. No matter how smart PubMed is, it can't always figure out what you mean – and even when it can, the number of results it spits

out is often overwhelming. In this chapter, we'll cover a couple of ways to make PubMed give you the results you want, not the results it thinks you might want.

8.2
What Is PubMed and How Does It Work?

Before searching PubMed, it is helpful to know a little about how it works. PubMed is the public interface to MEDLINE, the premier biomedical literature index. It's created by the National Library of Medicine, and each day, between 2,000 and 4,000 new citations are added to the database. It spans back to 1950, though the bulk of citations are from 1966 to the present, and contains well over 16 million records. As part of the NCBI Entrez system, it also interfaces with the rest of the databases in the Entrez system, including PubMed Central, a repository of freely available full-text journal articles; the NCBI Bookshelf, a set of full-text medical textbooks; OMIM (Online Mendelian Inheritance in Man), a genetic disease text; and dozens of genetics databases like GenBank, genomic sequencing databases, and more.

Though PubMed contains journal literature from more databases than MEDLINE, MEDLINE's the one it helps to know a little

M. Rethlefsen et al., *Internet Cool Tools for Physicians*
© Springer-Verlag Berlin Heidelberg 2009

8

about. MEDLINE is built around medical subject headings, a controlled vocabulary that gives MEDLINE its power. Because of medical subject headings, instead of having to think of all the possible relevant keywords to describe your topic, you can use one – the medical subject heading – and still get all the relevant articles. If you've searched MEDLINE via PubMed recently, you may not even realize that the medical subject headings are even there, much less a critical part of how PubMed is processing your search. It's all behind the scenes.

If you want to learn more about how PubMed and MEDLINE work, look for the excellent book, *MEDLINE: An Effective Guide to Searching in PubMed and Other Interfaces*, by Brian Katcher.

For each keyword that you enter into PubMed, PubMed will try to match it to a relevant medical subject heading. For example, let's say you are doing a search on heart attacks. If you type in the keywords heart attack, PubMed will translate that search into a query for the subject heading for heart attack, Myocardial Infarction. That way, even if the best articles on heart attacks don't use the phrase "heart attack" in the title or abstract, you'll still see them in your results list. You can always see how PubMed translates your search for you by looking in the Details tab underneath the search box.

After PubMed runs your search, it will give you the results it finds in reverse chronological order, the newest results put into the database always at the top. PubMed is updated everyday, Monday through Saturday, with new citations, meaning its data are much fresher than any other interface to MEDLINE.

8.3
PubMed Basics

There is more to PubMed than just the basic search box. Getting familiar with some of the other tools available to you can really help you soup up your PubMed experience.

8.3.1
Getting the Right Information

Using PubMed's keyword searching as is means that once in a while your search results may wind up completely unrelated to what you were looking for. Generally, this is a symptom of PubMed's poor mind-reading skills. Check the Details tab to see what PubMed did with your search – it may have misinterpreted your meaning or simply defaulted to searching a keyword.

Here's an example: if you search for the term *hrt* in PubMed, you may mean any number of things – hormone replacement therapy, heart rate turbulence, Heidelberg retinal tomography, etc. If you go to the Details tab, you'll see that PubMed didn't try to match your search term to a medical subject heading – it only searched hrt as a keyword. If you are really trying to get articles on hormone replacement therapy, then not only you are going to have to wade through a lot of articles on heart rate turbulence, but also you'll miss a lot of great articles on hormone replacement therapy. So, what can you do to turn this situation around? There are a couple of ways:

- Find the medical subject heading for your term
- Use the Related Articles feature
- Refrain from using abbreviations in the future

Though ceasing to use abbreviations will be a big help, the first two options are what will really improve your searching skills.

Finding a medical subject heading that matches your term is usually fairly simple. The easiest thing to do is to start with a quick keyword search and skim the results for an article you like. When you find one, click on the authors' names – this will take you into the "AbstractPlus" display. To see the medical subject headings, pull down the Display menu above the citation and select "Citation." Now, you'll see the medical subject headings below the abstract (Fig. 1). To search using one of those terms, you can copy and paste the term into the search box, or click on the term and select "PubMed" from the pop-up menu (Fig. 2).

> You can only find medical subject headings for articles that say [PubMed – indexed for MEDLINE] at the bottom of the citation. If it says [PubMed – as supplied by publisher] or [PubMed – in progress], you'll be out of luck. Those citations haven't been assigned subject headings yet.

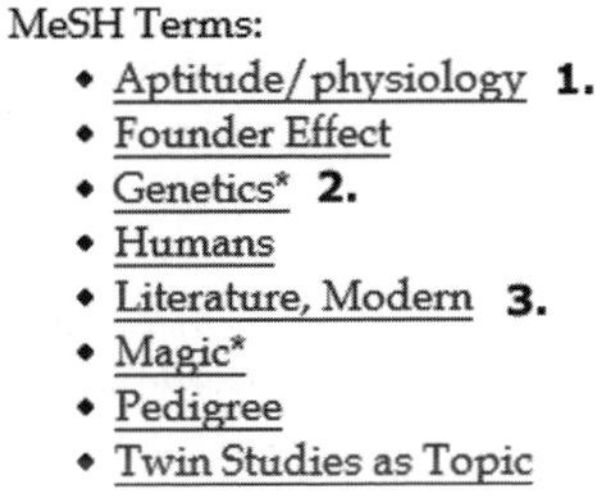

MeSH Terms:
- Aptitude/physiology **1.**
- Founder Effect
- Genetics* **2.**
- Humans
- Literature, Modern **3.**
- Magic*
- Pedigree
- Twin Studies as Topic

Fig. 1 Medical subject headings (MeSH terms) shown in Citation view. *1* Terms after slashes are called *sub-headings*. They represent an aspect of a particular heading and enable very specific searching. *2* Starred terms are major topic headings – main concepts for the article. *3* Unstarred terms are regular MeSH headings

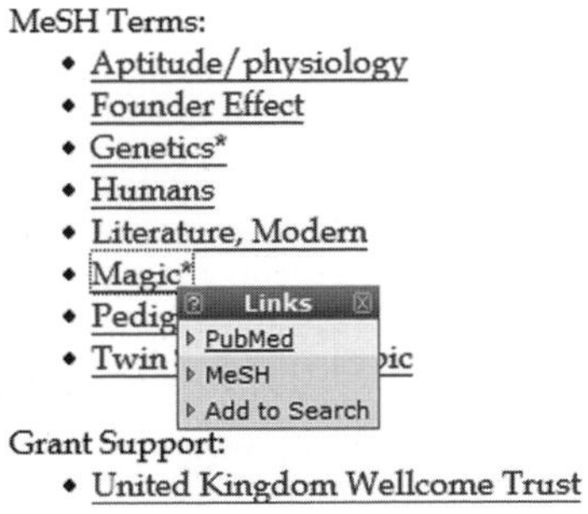

MeSH Terms:
- Aptitude/physiology
- Founder Effect
- Genetics*
- Humans
- Literature, Modern
- Magic*
- Pedig
- Twin

Links
▸ PubMed
▸ MeSH
▸ Add to Search

Grant Support:
- United Kingdom Wellcome Trust

Fig. 2 Clicking on a MeSH term in Citation view brings up the context menu. Click on PubMed to search for all articles indexed with that MeSH term

Using the Related Articles feature is even easier. Again, start by doing a quick search and finding an article you like. Once you find one, click on the Related Articles link to the right of the citation. PubMed will return a list of citations it thinks are related to your chosen article in relevancy ranked order.

> Using the Related Articles search is the only way to search for results ranked by relevancy when using PubMed. Remember, though, this means articles that are the most relevant could be from the 1960s. If you are looking for current articles only, you can sort the results by publication date using the Sort menu.

8.3.2
Using Limits

One of the biggest challenges in using PubMed is the huge number of results you get for most queries – no one has time to look through thousands of results, especially if you are using PubMed for clinical care. The fastest and easiest way to cut down on the number of results while improving their relevancy to your question is to use the Limits tab.

The Limits tab gives you a few quick check boxes to narrow your results down by:

- Type of article
- Age group
- Publication date
- Language

Limiting by publication date and language are fairly obvious limits, but most people aren't aware of the age group or publication type limits. The "type of article" limit is particularly useful for finding evidence-based information – you can quickly limit to clinical trials, randomized control trials, or systematic reviews. The age group limitations are especially nice for restricting your results to information on pediatric or geriatric populations – or to exclude them.

Tip. Are you searching PubMed to find patient care information? Try a tailored PubMed search interface to help you answer your clinical questions. PubMed provides a PICO (patient, intervention, comparison, outcome) search tool at http://pubmedhh.nlm.nih.gov/nlm/pico/piconew.html. It's designed for handheld computers, but works on a regular computer, too.

8.3.3
Using the Clipboard

The Clipboard is one of the most helpful features in PubMed. You can do multiple searches and keep your favorite results from each one – up to 500 citations for up to 8 h. To use the Clipboard: first, check the boxes next to the citations you like; second, use the Send to menu to select Clipboard. Your chosen citations will get stored in the Clipboard, plus will be marked in green in your next searches so you can easily skip over the results you've already seen. To get back to your saved citations, just click on the Clipboard tab.

8.3.4
The History Tab

Saving the citations you like is great, but often it would really be nice to get back to a search you

already did without having to type your terms in again. That's where the History tab can help. It keeps track of your searches over 8 h, so any search you already did is just two clicks away. To access your past searches, click on the History tab – once you're there, click on the number of results to rerun the search.

Thought that was cool? Well, the History tab has another great function. You can use it to combine your past searches together to make more complex searches. Let's say that you are doing a search looking for information on preventing obesity using physical activity. You started by doing a search for obesity prevention physical activity, and when that produced fewer results than you wanted, you did a second search for obesity prevention exercise. What you really want to do is look at the results of either of these searches at the same time. Here are the steps you would use:

1. Go to the History tab
2. Click clear to remove any search terms from the search box
3. Click on the search number corresponding to the obesity prevention physical activity search
4. On the pop-up Options menu, select AND
5. Click on the search number corresponding with the obesity prevention exercise search
6. On the pop-up Options menu, select OR
7. Click on the Go button

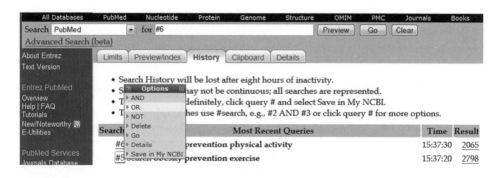

Fig. 3 Using the History tab to combine searches

Now your search results are broader – they include results from either individual search (Fig. 3).

A lot of times, you may do several similar searches in a row trying to figure out your best search terms. Use the NOT option in the History to remove older search results from your current search, or to remove citations already in your Clipboard from your current search (Clipboard results will always show as #0 in your History).

8.4
Even More PubMed Cool Tools

In the left-hand column of the PubMed display are a number of other tools that will kick your PubMed experience up a notch.

8.4.1
Clinical Queries

For patient care, the Clinical Queries feature provides a simple search interface for finding evidence-based resources to help answer clinical questions. Simply enter your search term; choose whether you want to look for etiology, diagnosis, clinical prediction guide, prognosis, or therapy studies; and select whether you want to have fewer (specific) results or more (sensitive) results. You will get fewer, more evidence-based results than doing a general search.

8.4.2
MeSH Database

Remember those medical subject heading things? The MeSH Database is a searchable database of those terms (MeSH stands for medical subject headings). With the MeSH Database, you can find medical subject headings that might be appropriate search terms for your query – this is especially useful if your keyword

searches aren't producing any good citations. Even better, you can get much fancier with your searching by using subheadings and major topic headings. You can even build your complex searches in the MeSH Database before searching in PubMed.

If you don't remember what subheadings and major topic headings are, check out the graphic in Sect. 8.3.1.

Using the MeSH Database can be tricky at first. Check out the great video tutorials provided on the MeSH Database home page (http://www.ncbi.nlm.nih.gov/sites/entrez?db=mesh) to get some pointers on using this cool tool.

8.4.3
My NCBI

The Entrez databases' personalization tool, My NCBI, is a must to try. My NCBI has several features that make searching PubMed much easier. To set up an account, click on My NCBI and then "register for an account." You'll need to choose a username and password and answer a security question. Though you don't have to provide an email address, it will be necessary if you want to use some of the features we'll cover in Chap. 10.

What are the benefits of having an account? One of the newest benefits is My NCBI Collections. With My NCBI Collections, you can store up to 100 sets of 1,500 citations each – permanently. Unlike the Clipboard, this isn't a temporary holding place, but one where you can access the research you need whenever you need it. To save citations in your Collection, you'll need to first send citations to the Clipboard (see Sect. 8.3.3). Once you have citations in the Clipboard, one of the Clipboard's Send to menu options will be My NCBI Collections. Simply name a new collection or choose an older collection. You can also use the Send to menu to save citations to a Collection directly from your search results page.

My NCBI also allows you to customize your PubMed display. You may have noticed that right above your search results, there are at least two tabs: All and Review. Those are filters – if you click on the Review tab, it will jump you directly to just the review articles in your set of results. With My NCBI, you can choose to add more of these filter tabs to your PubMed results. Let's say you are a pediatrician. One of the filters you might select could limit your results to the All Child age group. Any limit that you use frequently can be turned into a filter to make your searching less time consuming (Fig. 4).

To change your filters, go to My NCBI and select Filters from the left-hand menu. Once you are in the filters area, you can choose some common filters or click on the Browse tab to choose more filters. You can select up to five filters per database.

8.5
Finding Full-Text Articles

PubMed offers a dizzying array of options for finding full-text articles. Some of these options may be better for your practice than others, and some are certainly cheaper.

8.5.1
Pay per View

If you've searched PubMed a lot, you've probably seen the small, colorful graphics that often show up in the abstracts view. Often, they show a publisher's logo and the words "full text." These are publisher-supplied icons that link you directly to the full text of the article. PubMed has agreements with many different publishers, including all of the major medical publishers

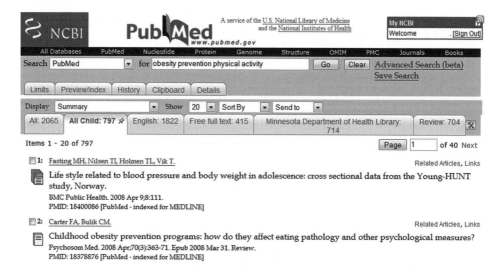

Fig. 4 Using the All Child filter added to PubMed display using Filters in My NCBI

like the American Medical Association, Elsevier, Springer, and Nature Publishing Group. These icons can be very deceiving – though they may promise full-text access to the articles you want, you may have to pay for the privilege of seeing them. Prices range from relatively inexpensive to simply prohibitive, depending on the publisher. Many publishers offer a day pass if you want to access multiple articles as well as single article pay per view.

8.5.2
Accessing Your Library's Resources Online

If you are affiliated with an academic institution or another medical library, your library may have set up a special way for you to access their online materials in PubMed. Libraries can create their own icons (called *link resolvers*) that will link you to their full-text articles online or to information about your library's print journal holdings. Often, libraries will provide a library-specific Web address for you to use.

If your library has established this kind of relationship (called *LinkOut*) with PubMed, you can also use My NCBI to help you access your full text. My NCBI gives you two options. You can choose to affiliate yourself with a library using the Outside Tool option, which will put your library's icon in each PubMed abstract, or you may be able to set up a My NCBI filter that limits your search to articles your library owns. To set up a filter, choose Libraries in the Filters' Browse page. All available libraries are listed alphabetically. Contact your library for more information on these tools.

8.5.3
Document Delivery

Though pay per view, library access, and freely available articles (see below) are the fastest options for getting journal articles, if you are willing to wait a few days, PubMed's document delivery options let you order articles from various document delivery services. If you are affiliated with a medical library, your library may provide Loansome Doc services to you for free or for a small fee (contact your library for help). You can also contract with a document delivery provider.

To set up your document delivery options, select Document Delivery from the left-hand menu in My NCBI. Listed are the various options for document delivery – Loansome Doc is the default. To find out more information about each of these services including cost, turnaround time, and delivery methods, follow the links to the various providers. Many (including Loansome Doc) require you to set up an account before using the service.

Even if you aren't affiliated with a medical library, many libraries provide document delivery services to the public via Loansome Doc. The library may charge a fee for service and for each article delivered, but these charges are often cheaper than pay-per-view services provided by publishers and document delivery services. Look for libraries serving "public users" in the Loansome Doc directory when registering for a Loansome Doc account (https://docline.gov/loansome/login.cfm).

To order articles from the document delivery service you set up in My NCBI, simply select the articles you wish to order. From the Send to menu, choose Order. You'll be taken to the document delivery provider Web site to complete your order.

8.5.4
Free Full Text

As the open access movement gains strength, more and more journals have some or all of their articles online for free. How can you find those articles easily? PubMed helps you out in a couple

8

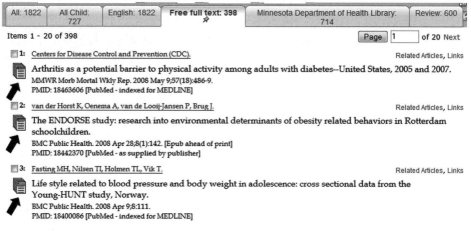

Fig. 5 Icons with *green bars* indicate that free full text is available for that article from the publisher. Icons with *green and orange bars* indicate that free full text is available in PubMed Central. PubMed Central full text may be directly from the publisher or may be a copy of the final manuscript as provided by the author(s)

of ways. For all of those articles it identifies as freely available, whether free from the publisher or in PubMed Central, PubMed displays the citation with one of two special icons in the summary view – a sheet of paper with a green bar denotes free full text from the publisher, and a sheet of paper with a green and orange bar denotes an article in PubMed Central. Using this visual cue, it's easy to scan a list of results for freely available articles.

PubMed Central is a repository for full-text articles, including articles from publishers and the manuscript versions of published articles that authors can submit. The manuscript versions will not have the formatting or sometimes even the editing that the published versions do.

To make it even easier, in the Limits tab, you can choose to limit to citations with links to free full-text articles. Remember those My NCBI Filters? Set up a filter to create a tab that will limit to free full-text articles – it's one of the quick picks (Fig. 5).

Though PubMed is pretty good at identifying those articles available free online, the links are limited to those journals whose publishers work with PubMed to set up links – and not all publishers do. To maximize your free full-text finding potential, you may want to try searching Google Scholar (http://scholar.google.com) or PubMed Gold (http://www.neurotransmitter.net/ftsearch.html) after you've tried your other PubMed options.

9.1
How Are Third-Party PubMed/MEDLINE Tools Possible?

The U.S. National Library of Medicine maintains a number of databases, including MEDLINE, a massive database of more than 16 million citations of biomedical literature, indexed by the NLM's controlled vocabulary of medical subject headings (MeSH). In addition to making MEDLINE (and other databases) available to be searched by anyone on the planet with a computer and an Internet connection through PubMed (http://www.pubmed.gov), they also make this data available through an API (details at http://www.ncbi.nlm.nih.gov/entrez/query/static/esoap_help.html).

9.2
What's an API?

An application programming interface (API) allows a program or database to be queried programmatically (by a computer or a program) instead of by a person through a Web-browser interface (like PubMed). This means that third parties (neither you nor the NLM) can write new tools that make use of the NLM's databases in ways that the NLM itself does not. Some of these tools can be extremely useful for specialized needs.

9.3
Search the Literature "Google-Style"

PubMed is best searched by using its native controlled vocabulary, MeSH, but many users are not familiar with it – so if a user enters search terms into PubMed as he would in Google, PubMed attempts to "map" (translate) these terms into MeSH, then execute the search. The results are returned in reverse chronological order with the most recent articles at the top.

With the global dominance of Google as the world's favorite search engine, there can be little doubt that many have wished for a PubMed interface that worked more like Google. ReleMed

9

(http://www.relemed.com), created by researchers at the University of Virginia School of Medicine, is just this sort of interface.

9.3.1
ReleMed

A search term entered into ReleMed, as in PubMed, is "mapped" to MeSH, but ReleMed uses a different set of tools to do the mapping and frequently produces better results (Fig. 1).

More important is how ReleMed sorts the search results. Where PubMed sorts result in reverse chronological order, ReleMed attempts to sort the search results the same way Google does, by relevance to your search. ReleMed accomplishes this based on the co-occurrence and proximity of search terms in the article's title, abstract, and MeSH terms in a process its creators call "sentence-level matching." In English, this means that articles where your search terms appear more frequently and closer to each other in the abstract and other elements of the citation will appear closer to the top of your search results.

When you see a result that interests you, you can even click the view PubMed record link to see that result's more complete record in PubMed.

9.3.2
Healia

Healia PubMed/MEDLINE Search (http://www.healia.com/healia/en/index.jsp?&mSp=pubmed)

doesn't reveal how (or if) it maps your search terms to MeSH, but like ReleMed, it attempts to sort search results by relevance. Although it doesn't disclose the mechanism by which its algorithm sorts for relevance, we can note that its relevance sorting differs from that of ReleMed. Healia PubMed/MEDLINE search also offers tabs to help quickly divide search results into Prevention, Causes/Risks, Symptoms, Diagnosis/Tests, and Treatment sections. This may help you narrow down your search results to the kinds of articles you most want to see. PubMed has an excellent Filters tab, but Healia's PubMed/MEDLINE interface places similar tools on a sidebar of the same screen as your search results, allowing you quick access to easily check off search refinements (Fig. 2).

9.4
Find the Right Author or Journal

9.4.1
PubFocus

Want to find the most influential or prolific authors for a particular topic or find out which journals have published the most about it? In its own words, PubFocus (http://www.pubfocus.com) "performs statistical analysis" of your query's results and gives them back to you with just this sort of information (Figs. 3–5).

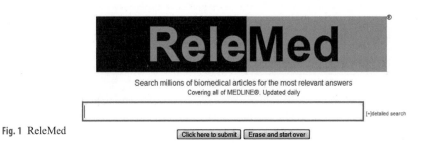

Fig. 1 ReleMed

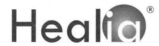

Fig. 2 Healia

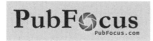

Fig. 3 PubFocus

9.4.2
PubReMiner

PubReMiner (http://bioinfo.amc.uva.nl/human-genetics/pubreminer) applies a slightly different sort of analysis of PubMed searches. When you enter as query into PubReMiner, it provides several of tables that count in descending order the calendar years in which articles fitting the query were most frequently published, the journals in which articles fitting the query were most frequently published, the authors whose articles most frequently fit the query, the words most often used in articles fitting the query, and the MeSH terms with which articles fitting the query are most frequently indexed (Fig. 6).

PubReMiner will also let you check off elements in the results tables and use them to further refine your search. When you've finished checking off the parts you want, PubReMiner will use them to produce a new, more complex query and run the query for you in PubMed. As the site itself points out, this sort of searching not only is useful in the creation and refinement of effective searches, but also can be applied to assist a clinician in selecting journals to which articles should best be submitted for publication, or can be used to identify experts in a particular field or specialty (Fig. 7).

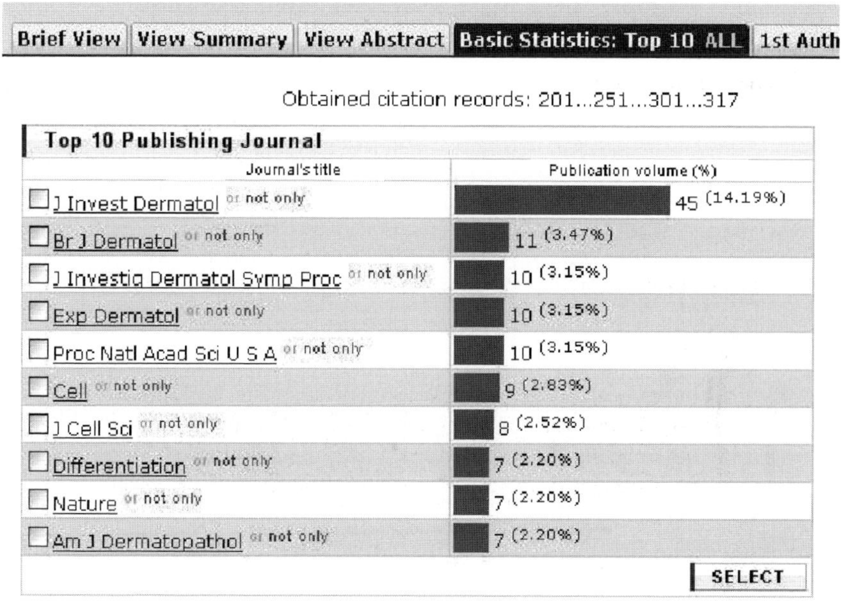

| Brief View | View Summary | View Abstract | **Basic Statistics: Top 10 ALL** | 1st Auth |

Obtained citation records: 201...251...301...317

Top 10 Publishing Journal	
Journal's title	Publication volume (%)
☐ J Invest Dermatol or not only	45 (14.19%)
☐ Br J Dermatol or not only	11 (3.47%)
☐ J Investig Dermatol Symp Proc or not only	10 (3.15%)
☐ Exp Dermatol or not only	10 (3.15%)
☐ Proc Natl Acad Sci U S A or not only	10 (3.15%)
☐ Cell or not only	9 (2.83%)
☐ J Cell Sci or not only	8 (2.52%)
☐ Differentiation or not only	7 (2.20%)
☐ Nature or not only	7 (2.20%)
☐ Am J Dermatopathol or not only	7 (2.20%)
	SELECT

Fig. 4 PubFocus Top Journals

t Basic Statistics: Top 10 ALL	1st Authors: Top 10 ALL	PI Authors: Top 10 ALL

Obtained citation records: 201...251...301...317

Top 10 Principal Investigators by AWF on all publications	
Author's name	Author's Weight Factor (AWF)
☐ **Cotsarelis G** or not only	142.35 (2.84%)
☐ **Fuchs E** or not only	73.76 (0.94%)
☐ **Hoffman Rm** or not only	62.27 (3.48%)
☐ **Barrandon Y** or not only	51.09 (1.26%)
☐ **Artandi Se** or not only	48.27 (0.31%)
☐ **Lavker Rm** or not only	47.51 (2.53%)
☐ **Morris Rj** or not only	39.98 (1.26%)
☐ **Blanpain C** or not only	36.71 (0.94%)
☐ **Sun Tt** or not only	33.59 (3.16%)
☐ **Nishimura Ek** or not only	33.56 (0.63%)
	SELECT

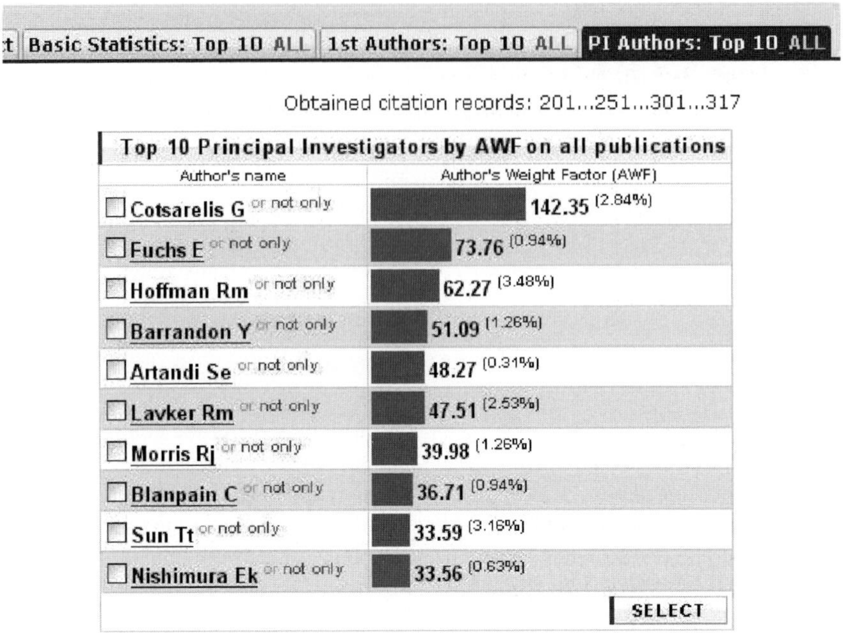

Fig. 5 PubFocus Top Authors

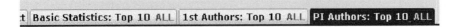

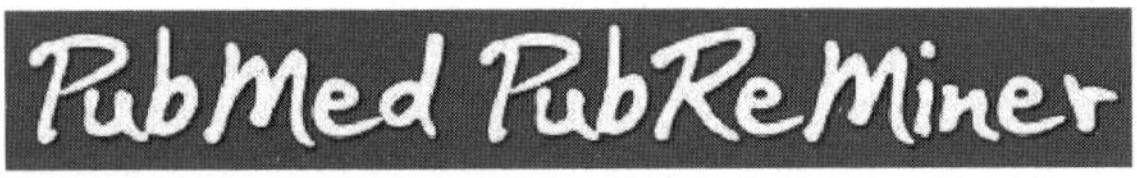

Fig. 6 PubReMiner

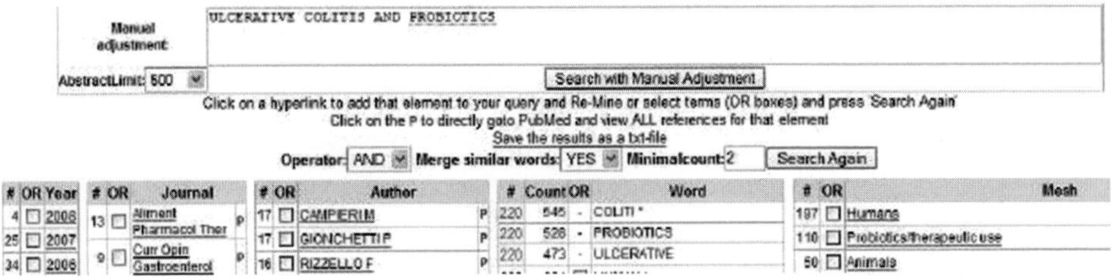

Manual adjustment:	ULCERATIVE COLITIS AND PROBIOTICS
AbstractLimit: 500	Search with Manual Adjustment

Click on a hyperlink to add that element to your query and Re-Mine or select terms (OR boxes) and press 'Search Again'
Click on the P to directly goto PubMed and view ALL references for that element
Save the results as a txt-file

Operator: AND | Merge similar words: YES | Minimalcount: 2 | Search Again

# OR	Year	# OR	Journal	# OR	Author		# Count OR	Word	# OR	Mesh
4 ☐	2008	13 ☐	Aliment Pharmacol Ther	17 ☐	CAMPIERI M	P	220 545 -	COLITI *	197 ☐	Humans
25 ☐	2007			17 ☐	GIONCHETTI P	P	220 526 -	PROBIOTICS	110 ☐	Probiotics/therapeutic use
34 ☐	2006	9 ☐	Curr Opin Gastroenterol	16 ☐	RIZZELLO F	P	220 473 -	ULCERATIVE	50 ☐	Animals

Fig. 7 PubReMiner

9.4.3
JANE

JANE (http://biosemantics.org/jane/) is a "journal/article name estimator." Not sure to which journals you best should submit your article or looking for an appropriate peer reviewer? Paste your article's contents into JANE and JANE will "compare your document to millions of documents in MEDLINE to find the best matching journals or authors" (Fig. 8).

If the idea of JANE appeals to you, be sure also to try out eTBLAST (http://invention. swmed.edu/etblast/etblast.shtml/), a similar service with some additional refinement tools and access to science databases other than those of the National Library of Medicine.

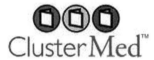

Fig. 10 GoPubMed

9.5
Get a Communal Evaluation... or Help Create One

Digg (http://www.digg.com) is a popular Web site on which members communally rate and comment on news items. BioWizard (http://www. biowizard.com) takes the example of Digg and runs with it, allowing you to search for and submit items from PubMed with a single click to a collaborative evaluation and discussion platform where other biomedical researchers can rate and/ or comment on the article. BioWizard also offers Web pages and RSS feeds (See Chap. 11 for more information on RSS feeds) listing articles submitted and highly rated by users in many categories of biomedical research. While there are numerous sites that utilize the Digg model to allow clinicians to collaboratively evaluate online items, BioWizard is the only one (at the time of this writing) which limits submissions to items that can be found in PubMed, insuring that all items communally evaluated in BioWizard are from the professional literature, not popular or consumer-oriented media (Fig. 9).

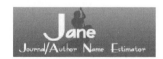

Fig. 8 JANE

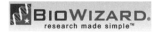

Fig. 9 BioWizard

Fig. 11 ClusterMed

9.6
Browse Search Results by "Clusters"

9.6.1
GoPubMed

GoPubMed (http://www.gopubmed.com/) is named for its ability to utilize Gene Ontology, but what we like best about it is the way it analyzes each search and "clusters" elements of metadata found in the search results, allowing you to see (and filter for) trends of authors, journals, countries, and MeSH terms. GoPubMed will also produce a list of MeSH terms strongly related to your search and produce a frequency analysis of a given MeSH term in the literature your search returns over time (Fig. 10).

9.6.2
ClusterMed

ClusterMed (http://clustermed.info) also "clusters" your search results with a navigation tool in the left sidebar, allowing you to browse them by authors, authors' institutional affiliations, MeSH, or words appearing frequently in titles and abstracts of articles returned by your search (Fig. 11).

9

9.7
Enhance Your Browser

The NLM Toolbar (http://nlm.ourtoolbar. com/) was created by Guus van den Brekel, a Dutch medical librarian. This toolbar embeds a plethora of useful tools in your Internet Explorer or Firefox Web browser, including buttons to jump you straight to particular resources offered by the National Library of Medicine, the ability to search any of the NLM's databases regardless of what site your browser currently has loaded, quick access to all RSS feeds offered by the NLM, and many more (Fig. 12).

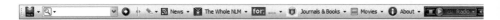

Fig. 12 NLM Toolbar

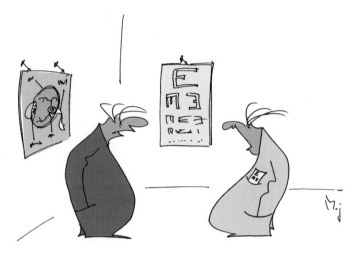

How much are you willing to bid on eBay for your new cornea?

Email Alerts

10

10.1
Email Alerts

Email alerts are one of the easiest ways to receive new information on topics of interest to you. Most journals offer email alerting services for tables of contents, early release papers, and news. Many databases, Web sites, and newspapers also provide email alerting tools. Since email is already a critical tool for most physicians, it's a convenient way to access the latest information you want to read.

10.2
PubMed (http://www.pubmed.gov)

PubMed is one of the best places to create email alerts. For any PubMed search that you do, you can create a personalized email update. This is particularly helpful for searches on a specific topic or by a particular author. To create an email alert, you will need a My NCBI account (see Sect. 8.4.3 for more information on My NCBI).

The first step in creating a PubMed email alert is to perform a PubMed search (see Sect. 8.3 for tips on searching PubMed). As soon as you perform a search in PubMed, a Save Search link appears to the right of the search box. Follow this link to create your email alert. Note: If you don't have a My NCBI account, you will be prompted to register for one.

Once you've logged into My NCBI, you can choose a name for your search and whether you'd like to receive email updates. If you select yes, extra options appear below. These options allow you to choose how often you want to receive your updates (daily, weekly, and monthly options are available), what day of the week or month you want to receive your updates, the format of your updates (plain text or Web-based format), and the maximum number of items to send per update. Once you pick your selections, click on OK to start receiving your email alerts (Fig. 1).

M. Rethlefsen et al., *Internet Cool Tools for Physicians*
© Springer-Verlag Berlin Heidelberg 2009

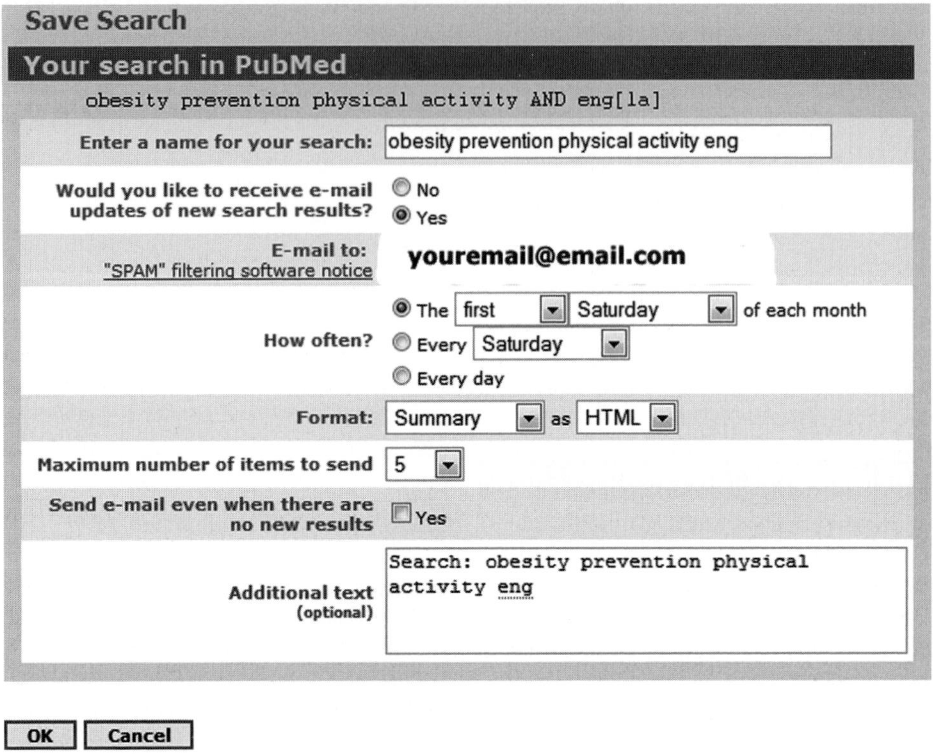

10

Save Search

Your search in PubMed

obesity prevention physical activity AND eng[la]

Enter a name for your search: | obesity prevention physical activity eng |

Would you like to receive e-mail
updates of new search results?
○ No
◉ Yes

E-mail to:
"SPAM" filtering software notice   **youremail@email.com**

How often?
◉ The | first ▾ | Saturday ▾ | of each month
○ Every | Saturday ▾ |
○ Every day

Format: | Summary ▾ | as | HTML ▾ |

Maximum number of items to send | 5 ▾ |

Send e-mail even when there are
no new results
☐ Yes

Additional text
(optional)
| Search: obesity prevention physical
activity eng |

[OK]   [Cancel]

Fig. 1 Setting up an email alert through PubMed's My NCBI service

To avoid being overwhelmed by the number of results you receive per email, test out your search to see how many items you'll receive per month. The easiest way to do this is to perform your search and use the Limits tab (see Sect. 8.3.2 for help using the Limits tab). From the Added to PubMed in the Last menu, choose 30, 60, or 90 days to get a feel for how many items get added per month in your topic. If the numbers you see are too much, try narrowing your search down using some Limits like language and type of article, or by making your search terms more specific.

10.3
What Are My Other Options for Email Alerts?

If you have access to subscription-based biomedical literature databases, you have even more options for email alerts. Nearly all of the fee-based and subscription-based databases offer email alerting services, including Scopus, ISI Web of Science, Ovid SP databases (Current Contents, MEDLINE, EMBASE, etc.), EMBASE. com, and many others. Look for saved search or email alerting options.

HighWire Press (http://highwire.stanford. edu), the electronic journals publisher that publishes many of the major medical journals online, including New England Journal of Medicine, JAMA, and BMJ, has a freely available search alerting service. Though the search is restricted to HighWire Press' electronic journals, you can choose to search the full text of journal articles when setting up your alerts. This means that though you don't have the benefits of a controlled vocabulary like you would in PubMed, you can broaden your search to the full content of articles, thus potentially picking up additional resources.

To set up a search alert at HighWire Press, you will need to create a personal account. On the main HighWire Press page, follow the link to create a free account. Once you've created the account and verified your email address, perform a search for a topic or author of your choice. Click on the Create Alert button to set up the email update. You can choose to only receive updates from particular journals, all HighWire Press content, or even all PubMed content.

Scopus, ISI Web of Science, and HighWire Press, in addition to offering email updates for searches, also provide citation alerting services. When a particular article of your choice is cited by any other article, you would receive an alert. This type of alert is very useful for tracking citations to your publications and for discovering new articles you may have missed in a regular literature search.

10.4
What About Tables of Contents via Email?

One of the most important ways of keeping up to date is by browsing and reading general and specialty medical journals in your field. As more personal and institutional journal subscriptions turn to online-only access, it's important to continue to browse and read these titles, even with-

out the journal physically in front of you. This is where tables of contents email alerting services help. With email alerts from publishers and databases, you can still have the serendipity of discovering new material.

10.5
How Do I Sign Up for Email Tables of Contents?

Nearly every publisher of biomedical journals supplies an email alerting service for tables of contents freely, even though you may not have a subscription to the full content. If you do not have access through either an individual or an institutional subscription, most publishers have pay-per-view or pay-by-day systems in place.

If you are affiliated with a library (public, academic, or hospital), you may be able to request copies of articles via interlibrary loan. You may also be able to locate manuscripts or self-archived versions free through PubMed Central (http://pubmedcentral.nih.gov) or Google Scholar (http://scholar.google.com). See Sect. 8.5 for more options for accessing full-text articles.

10.5.1
ScienceDirect (http://www.sciencedirect.com)

ScienceDirect is the e-journal publishing platform for Reed Elsevier, one of the largest scientific, technical, and medical publishers. Even without institutional access, anyone visiting the ScienceDirect Web site can set up email alerts by topic or for journal tables of contents. To sign up for alerts on ScienceDirect, you will need to create an account. Set up an account by following the Not Registered link in the top right of the screen. Registration at ScienceDirect requires a name, email address, location (country), and password. Once you've created an account, you can use the Alerts tab to create your alerts.

10

To access full-text articles without a subscription, ScienceDirect offers fee-based 24-h online access and downloading.

10.5.2
HighWire Press

HighWire Press publishes many major medical and scientific electronic journals, including those produced by the American Medical Association, BMJ Publishing Group, American Academy of Pediatrics, American Society for Microbiology, and many more. A large number of HighWire Press titles have some free content; a few are open access. A complete list of available HighWire Press titles and their full-text availability is available at http://highwire.stanford.edu/lists/allsites.dtl.

Many HighWire Press titles allow you to set up email notifications directly from the journal's Web page. To save some time, if you want to subscribe to email alerts for more than one HighWire Press title, visit the HighWire Press Web site (http://highwire.stanford.edu) and create a personal account. From there, go to the Alerts tab. Under My eTOC Alerts, select Add. From the complete list of HighWire Press titles that appears, you can choose to subscribe to full tables of contents, notification of new tables of contents, articles published ahead of print where available, announcements, and future tables of contents. After you select your titles, click on the Update eTOC Alerts button to save your preferences.

10.5.3
More Publishers

Wiley InterScience (http://www.interscience.wiley.com) and SpringerLink (http://springerlink.metapress.com) are other scientific, technical, and medical electronic journal publishers with email alerting services. Both require registration.

10.6
What About Journals That Don't Have Email Alerts?

Though the e-journal publishers listed above comprise a large majority of biomedical journals, there are some journals from smaller publishers that may not have email alerting tools. Luckily, by using PubMed's My NCBI email updates, you can get tables of contents emailed to you from any one of the 4,500 biomedical journals PubMed indexes. In fact, you can use My NCBI to set up all your email alerts at once, saving you the hassle of creating multiple accounts across the many e-journal publishing platforms.

Benefits of Using PubMed's My NCBI for Tables of Contents Alerting

- Only need to create a single account
- Can subscribe to tables of contents of 4,500 different biomedical journals
- Email alerts have links back to PubMed for easier access to freely available manuscripts from PubMed Central, links to library or publisher resources, and PubMed tools

Drawbacks of Using PubMed's My NCBI for Tables of Contents Alerting

- Delay between release of articles on publisher site and entry into PubMed can be up to 3–6 months depending on the journal, though usually the delay is only a few days to a week
- You may not receive the entire tables of contents in one day due to delays in data entry

10.7
How Do I Create Email Alerts for Tables of Contents in PubMed?

In PubMed, go to the Limits tab. In the Search by Journal bar, select Add Journal. Enter in a journal's full title or an abbreviation. Select the correct journal name from the list that appears. If you want to create a single alert for more than one journal title, simply click on Add Another Journal, and repeat as desired. Click on Go when you've chosen your journals (Fig. 2).

If you only wish to get articles on certain topics from a particular journal, you can add search terms to the PubMed search box before clicking on Go.

After you've clicked on Go, the search will run and the Save Search link will appear to the right of the search box. Follow this link to create your email alert. If you don't have a My NCBI account, you will be prompted to register for one.

Once you've logged into My NCBI, select yes to set up your email alert. Choose how often you want to receive your updates (daily, weekly, and monthly options are available), what day of the week or month you want to receive your updates, the format of your updates (plain text or Web-based format), and the maximum number of items to send per update. Once you pick your selections, click on OK to start receiving your email alerts.

Some journals, particularly news-heavy weekly titles like Science, Nature, and BMJ, will produce well over 50 new items per week. If you are subscribing to a weekly title, make sure that you select a high maximum number of items to receive per update and pick a weekly or daily frequency to receive alerts.

10.8
More Content, More Alerting Tools

10.8.1
Google Alerts

Obviously, not everything that you want to stay up to date with is in biomedical journals. For more general types of information, you can use the Google Alerts service (http://www.google.com/alerts) to keep tabs on new Web content. Pop in a keyword or two, select a frequency for receiving your email alerts, and enter an email address. After that, anytime something new is published on the Web on your topic, you'll be notified.

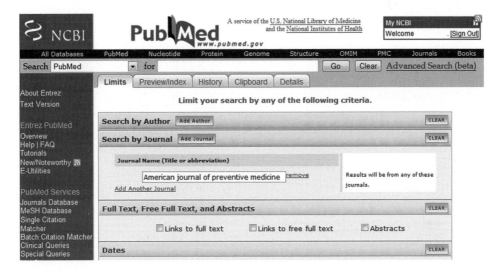

Fig. 2 Using the Limits tab's Search by Journal field to set up an email alert for a journal table of contents

10

Most of us want to know what's being said about us on the Web. Try setting up a Google Alert for your name or your institution's name to find out what people are saying.

The default type of search in a Google Alert is comprehensive – that means that you'll get notified about new content from most of Google's services, including general Web search, news, videos, and blogs (see Chap. 15 for information about blogs). You can change the type of content you want to receive in the Type menu option.

10.8.2
Google News Alerts

Though Google News is one of the options in the regular Google Alerts tool, you can also set up news alerts directly through Google News (http://news.google.com). Google News is Google's specialty news search engine covering approximately 4,500 international news publications. Google News, like Google, is also available in country-specific versions (e.g., http://news.google.de for Germany or http://news.google.se for Sweden), though each country's number of news sources will vary. The complete list of available Google News versions is at the bottom of the main Google News page.

The news on the main Google page is customized for each country, and a few country-specific Google News versions may not have a News Alerts option. For those that do, look for a News Alerts link and envelope icon after you perform a search for your topic. You can use several special searching tricks to create a personalized news alert using the Advanced News Search page linked from the right of the search box. Most importantly, the Advanced Search includes limits by publication source and location to limit to your search and alerts to a specific locale (Fig. 3).

You can bypass the Advanced Search page using special commands. To limit to a particular location, use location: plus a U.S. state or country; to limit to a particular source, use source: plus a partial or complete source name. If you use a complete source name, put it in quotation marks.

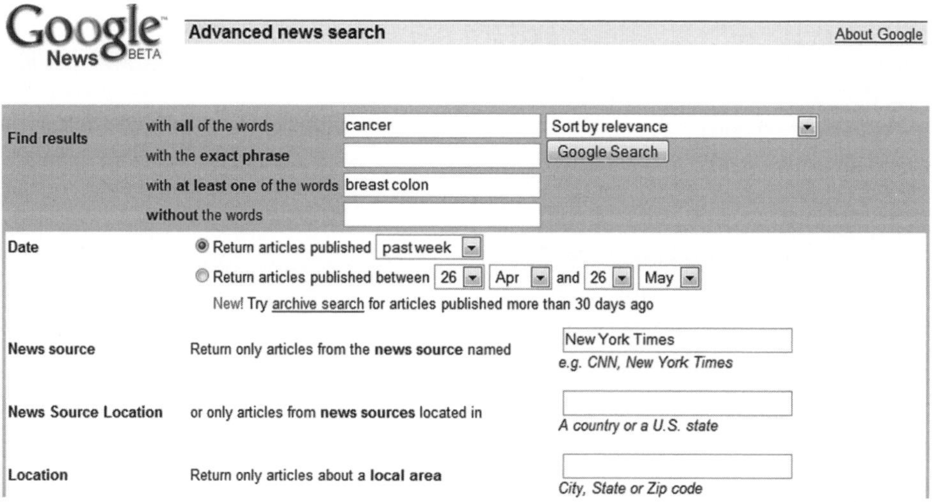

Fig. 3 Using the Advanced Search in Google News to limit a news search to a particular publication – here, the New York Times

Example 1:

basketball source:"new york"

Example 2:

president location:germany

Because the Google News databases are constantly updated, News Alerts offer an as-it-happens alerting option so you can get up to the minute information. You can set up as many as 1,000 alerts.

If you have a Yahoo! email address, you can also set up news alerts at Yahoo! News (http://beta.alerts.yahoo.com). Yahoo! can also alert you to stock value changes, airline flight specials, and more. You can also send your Yahoo! alerts to a mobile phone or to Yahoo! Messenger, Yahoo's instant messaging tool. Yahoo! allows up to 100 alerts per email account.

If your favorite Web page doesn't have an email alerting service to let you know when changes are made, try a Web monitoring tool like watchthatpage.com. Web monitoring tools will let you know whenever the content of any Web page changes.

I'm here to excise the optical drive ...

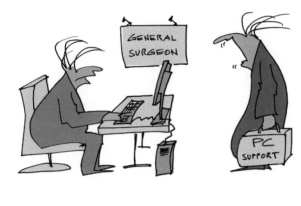

11

Core Messages

›   RSS is a syndication technology that can help you stay efficiently up to date on almost any kind of information.

›   Use an aggregator as a central location for reading your feed subscriptions.

›   Feeds can be found from many sources, including PubMed, MedWorm, blogs, and journal tables of contents.

11.1
What Is RSS?

The acronym "RSS" can stand for "rich site summary," "RDF (resource description framework) site summary," or "really simple syndication." RSS is an XML (extensible markup language) document format used to syndicate information on the Web.

I sometimes see references to "Atom feeds." Is Atom a kind of RSS feed?

Atom, like RSS, is an XML-based syndication format. It does have significant differences from RSS, but these differences should be imperceptible to the average user. In this chapter, everything said about RSS can also be applied to Atom.

More simply, the Internet is full of useful information that is constantly updating. In an attempt to keep up with this onslaught of information, Dr. Brown might check MedScape Today (http://www.medscape.com/medscapetoday) about once per day to see if there are any news headlines his cardiology patients are going to be asking him about. Dr. Green has four physician blogs that he reads and tries to remember to check them everyday…or even multiple times each day. Dr. Blue, an obstetric surgeon, makes a monthly stop in to her hospital's medical library to flip through the tables of contents in the core journals of her specialty to see if there are any new articles about obstetric hemorrhage she should read.

These important current awareness activities are, let's face it, incredibly time consuming. RSS can make each of these activities faster, more efficient, and more pleasant. Rather than you having to go to these Web sites to see what's new, RSS can deliver it directly to you. What if, instead of Dr. Brown having to visit MedScape Today every day, he could tell a program that he'd like to be notified every time there's a new story on MedScape Today that he can either choose to read or just discard? What if Dr. Green could instruct a program to grab all the new posts from his favorite blogs so he could check them all at once, in one place, quickly and easily? What if Dr. Blue could

M. Rethlefsen et al., *Internet Cool Tools for Physicians*
© Springer-Verlag Berlin Heidelberg 2009

11

automatically be informed every time there was a new article on obstetric hemorrhage in her core journals without ever having to go to the library to look through tables of contents? RSS makes it possible. RSS delivers this information to the physician instead of the physician having to go out and find it.

11.2
What's an Aggregator?

An aggregator (sometimes called a "feed reader," a "news reader," or just a "reader") is the tool where the information you want is delivered so you can efficiently receive and review it in one place.

There are several kinds of aggregators you can choose from. Some aggregators are standalone programs that you can install on a computer, some are a part of other programs (Outlook 2007, Internet Explorer 7+, and Firefox 2+ all have aggregators built into them), and some programs can have aggregator functionality added to them by installing a free or inexpensive add-on. Outlook 2000 or Outlook 2003, for example, can be given aggregator capabilities by installing RSS Popper (http://rsspopper. blogspot.com/2004/10/home.html), BlogBot for Outlook (http://blogbot.com/out/), Inclue! (http:// www.inclue.com/home/), or IntraVnews (http:// www.intravnews.com/).

Despite all of these options, we'll focus here on Web-based aggregators like Google Reader (http://www.google.com/reader/) because most physicians need to use multiple computers, and a Web-based aggregator allows you to access your feeds from any computer in the same way that Web-based email (like Hotmail, Gmail, Yahoo! email, or Outlook Web Access) allows you to access your email from any computer. For the sake of simplicity, we'll use Google Reader in the examples, but you'll be able to easily transition to another aggregator later if you prefer.

Need help figuring out which aggregator would be right for your needs? We think that Bloglines (http://www.bloglines.com/) and Google Reader (http://www.google.com/reader/) are good bets for most users, but you can use these resources to help you explore other options:

- RSS Compendium: RSS Readers (http:// allrss.com/rssreaderswebbased.html)
- A directory of RSS Aggregators (http:// www.aggcompare.com/)

First, go to Google Reader (http://www. google.com/reader/) and follow the instructions there to sign up for a free account. If you already have a Google Account for another Google service, you can use it to access Google Reader

11.3
Finding and Subscribing to Feeds

Next you'll want to tell Google Reader what sorts of things you want to be kept up to date on.

Click on the "Add subscription" link in the upper left corner of Google Reader. You we'll be prompted to provide the URL (Web address) of a feed (Fig. 1).

If you don't know the feed's URL offhand, you can ask Google Reader to search for it. Search for the MedScape Today feed by typing medscape and clicking the "Add" button. Google Reader will check through its database of all the feeds that all of its readers are subscribed to and suggest feeds that might be a match. When you see your match, click the "Subscribe" button to receive notification of all new items from that feed (Fig. 2).

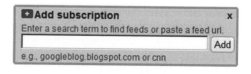

Fig. 1 Add a subscription to a feed by entering a feed's URL or a search term

Medscape Today Headlines

Latest medical news, articles, and features from **Medscape** Today
http://www.medscape.com/cx/rssfeeds/medscapetoday.xml - 0.0 posts per week

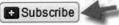

Fig. 2 Click on the Subscribe button to subscribe to a feed

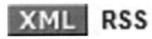

Fig. 3 RSS feed icons located on MedScape Today Web page

Fig. 4 The standard RSS feed icon

If Google Reader can't find the feed you're looking for, you can go look for it on the site whose feed you want to subscribe to. At the time of this writing, you can look on MedScape Today's (http://www.medscape.com/medscape-today) right sidebar, and find links to its feeds by looking for "XML" or "RSS" (Fig. 3)

Right click on either of these and choose "Copy Link Location" or "Copy Shortcut," then go back to Google Reader, click "Add subscription," and paste in the feed URL and click "Add."

Not every site will advertise its feed in the same way. Although many sites are now using a "standard" RSS icon, others may advertise it with "RSS," "XML," "Subscription," "Feed," or "Syndication" (Fig. 4).

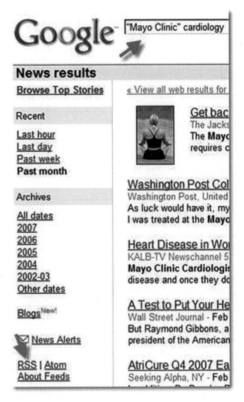

Fig. 5 Finding an RSS feed for a Google News search mayocardiology.jpg

11.4
What Sorts of Feeds Might Be Most Useful?

11.4.1
News from Media Outlets

Services like Google News (http://news.google.com/), Yahoo News (http://news.yahoo.com/), and Topix (http://www.topix.com/) crawl the Web collecting stories from the Web sites of newspapers, television stations, and other news media sources. You can search any of these for stories that interest you. If, for instance, you're interested in news stories about cardiology at the Mayo Clinic, you could go to Google News and search for "Mayo Clinic" cardiology, then click on the RSS link on the lower left of the page to get the URL to subscribe to (Fig. 5).

11

11.4.2
PubMed Search

Take the example of Dr. Blue at the beginning of this chapter. She wants to know any time one of the core journals in her field (obstetric surgery) has an article about hemorrhage. To accomplish this, she can run a search in PubMed, then subscribe to a feed for any new items that meet the criteria of that search.

First, go to PubMed (http://www.pubmed.gov), type "hemorrhage" into the search field, and click on the Limits tab (see Sect. 8.3.2 for more information on PubMed's Limits tab).

On the Limits tab, click "Add Journal" and start typing in the names of the journals (PubMed will cleverly offer you completed names of journals to choose from, so you never have to type very much) (Fig. 6).

Now, you'll need to scroll down to the bottom of the screen and click the Go button to run the search.

If you'd like to be able to click on articles in your RSS feeds and jump straight to the full-text article as often as possible, you'll probably want to visit your medical library. Your medical librarian can help you (or show you how to) create and subscribe to a search (perhaps using PubMed LinkOut, EBSCO MEDLINE, or OVID) that will maximize the number of full-text articles you can access directly from your RSS feeds by utilizing the resources. Your medical librarian can also assist you with searches that are more complex than this simple example to help make sure the items you receive in your aggregator are just the sorts of articles you're interested in seeing.

Search by Journal **Add Journal**

Journal Name (Title or abbreviation)

American journal of obstetrics and gyneco remove

Obstetrics and gynecology remove

Surgery, gynecology & obstetrics remove

British journal of obstetrics and gynaecol remove

Clinical obstetrics and gynecology remove

Add Another Journal

Fig. 6 Limiting a PubMed search to selected journals in the Limits tab

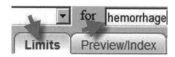

Fig. 7 (Google news search)

11.4.3
Your Favorite Blogs

Virtually every blog has an RSS feed. See Chap. 14 for details on finding healthcare blogs that suit your interests and preferences.

11.4.4
Tables of Contents (TOCs) from Publishers

Many journal publishers offer feeds to keep readers updated when new tables of contents or other materials are available. The New England Journal of Medicine has a page full of RSS feeds (http://content.nejm.org/rss/), as do the journals of the American Medical Association (http://pubs.ama-assn.org/misc/rssfeed.dtl), the Annals of Internal Medicine (http://www.annals.org/rss/), BMJ (http://www.bmj.com/rss/), and The Lancet (http://www.thelancet.com/rss).

Some journals don't offer feeds yet. When you encounter a journal you'd like to have in your aggregator but the journal doesn't appear to offer a feed for its table of contents, you have two options:

Option A. Create a feed for the journal in PubMed.

1. Navigate to PubMed (http://www.pubmed.gov/)
2. Click on the Limits tab
3. Click the Add Journal button
4. Type in the name of the journal
5. Scroll down to the bottom of the page and click the Go button
6. Go to the Send to drop-down menu and select RSS Feed
7. At Limit Items if more than, choose 50
8. Click Create Feed button

9. Click on the orange XML button and copy and paste the URL from the address bar into your favorite aggregator

Option B. Check MedWorm to see if MedWorm has a feed for the journal.

1. Navigate to MedWorm (http://www.medworm.com)
2. Click on the Publications Directory link (http://www.medworm.com/rss/medicine-category.php)
3. Click on the specialty or field in which the journal you're looking for would be categorized
4. Click on the name of the journal
5. At the top of this page will be several buttons including the standard, square orange feed button and a handful of buttons that will allow you to add the feed to one of several Web-based aggregators with a single click (Fig. 8).

11.4.5
MedWorm Search

Created by an English software developer who is married to a physician, MedWorm (http://www.medworm.com) monitors over 5,000 feeds from a broad variety of sources for health information and provides powerful tools for browsing, searching, or subscribing to the contents of these feeds. Even more important, the results of any search can be output as an RSS feed you can subscribe to. This means that when MedWorm discovers a new item that matches your search criteria, you're informed about it and given a link to read it. MedWorm also allows you to search subsets of feeds, including feeds from mainstream health news sources, feeds from

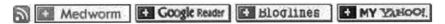

Fig. 8 RSS subscription buttons in MedWorm

11

consumer health information sources, feeds from medical journals, feeds from healthcare organizations, feeds from the medical blogosphere (see Chap. 15 for more information on blogs), and healthcare podcast feeds (see Chap. 13 for information on podcasts).

There are three radio buttons beneath MedWorm's search field, any words, all words, and exact phrase:

1. **Any words.** By default, the any words radio button is selected when you first load the main page of MedWorm in your Web browser. Having this radio button selected tells MedWorm that your search results must contain at least one of the words you're searching for.
2. **All words.** The all words radio button tells MedWorm that you only want results that contain all of the words you're searching for.
3. **Exact phrase.** The exact phrase radio button tells MedWorm that you only want to see search results that contain exactly the characters in the exact sequence you typed into the search field. Posts that don't contain exactly this string of characters in this sequence, even if they contain something very similar, will not appear in the results of this search.

MedWorm also makes use of powerful search operators (Note: For best results, select the any words radio button before using these operators.):

- " " (quotation marks)
  - A phrase that is enclosed within double quote (" ") characters matches only rows that contain the phrase exactly as it was typed (see notes on "exact phrase" radio button above).
- +
  - A plus sign (+) before a word indicates to MedWorm that the word must be present in every result returned.
- −
  - The leading minus sign (-) indicates that the word must not appear in any search result returned.

- *
  - The asterisk is the truncation or wildcard character in MedWorm. For example, if we were to search MedWorm for cardi*, we'd receive search results that included cardiac, cardiology, cardiologist, etc.
- ( )
  - Parentheses group words into subexpressions. For example, if we were to search +("mayo clinic" "cleveland clinic" "johns hopkins") + cardiology, this query will produce results that contain the exact phrase "cardiology" AND either "mayo clinics," "cleveland clinic," or "johns hopkins."
- ~
  - This operator (the tilde) is sort of like the − (minus sign) operator, but not as emphatic. A search term with this operator in front of it will not be excluded from results returned, but the term's presence will not be considered in the sorting of results by relevance. It sort of de-emphasizes the search term without absolutely removing the term from your results.

Try these operators out and you'll find you can generate very specific results.

11.4.6
Creating Feeds for Pages that Do Not Offer Them

Sometimes you'll want to be kept up to date on changes to a particular Web page that doesn't offer a feed and is not indexed by PubMed. In these cases, you can use a class of free Web services that are frequently called "scrapers." These scrapers are programs that will go to a Web page in regular intervals, look for new information, and output this information as an RSS feed that you can subscribe to. Feed43 (http://feed43.com/) is probably the most powerful of these and definitely the tool we'd recommend for users who enjoy some familiarity with HTML, but it also has the steepest and most difficult learning curve.

For beginners, try PonyFish (http://www.pony-fish.com/) or Page2RSS (http://page2rss.com/). If neither of those will meet your needs, try Dapper (http://www.dapper.net/), Feedity (http://www.feedity.com/), FeedYes (http://www.feedyes.com/), or WotzWot RSSxl (http://www.wotzwot.com/rssxl.php).

11.5
Manipulating Feeds

A number of free services will let you combine multiple feeds into one, or filter feeds for just the items you want to see.

11.5.1
Filtering Feeds

For example, say you want to monitor news items from WebMD's main RSS feed (http://rssfeeds.webmd.com/rss/rss.aspx?RSSSource=RSS_PUBLIC), but you really only want to see the items that mention cancer. For this example, we'll use FeedRinse (http://feedrinse.com/):

1. Navigate to FeedRinse (http://feedrinse.com/)
2. Register to get a free account
3. Click Add Feeds button

4. Under Enter your subscription URL(s) here, paste in your feed URL (http://rssfeeds.webmd.com/rss/rss.aspx?RSSSource=RSS_PUBLIC) and click the Import button
5. Click the Set up rules button
6. Use the drop-down menus to instruct Feed-Rinse to allow the post if any of the following conditions are met: post contains cancer
7. Click the Save changes button
8. Obtain the URL for the filtered feed that shows only posts in which the word "cancer" appears by clicking on the RSS icon to the left of the feed's name. FeedRinse will also offer to help you quickly and easily subscribe to this filtered feed in many popular Web-based aggregators (Figs. 9 and 10).

11.5.2
Combining Feeds

For example, let's say we've already filtered feeds from WebMD news and MedScape news to just show posts that mention cancer and would like to combine the two feeds into a single feed we'll call "Cancer News":

1. Still in FeedRinse (http://feedrinse.com/), click Create a channel
2. Give your channel a name ("Cancer News") and click the Continue button

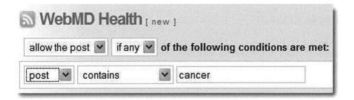

Fig. 9 Using the drop-down menus to instruct FeedRinse to allow the post when certain conditions are met

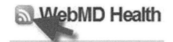

Fig. 10 Click the RSS icon to obtain the filtered RSS feed's URL or Web address

3. Select the two feeds you want to combine and click Save changes (Fig. 11)
4. On the your channels tab, you'll now see a channel called "Cancer News." Click the icon to the left of this title to quickly and easily subscribe to this feed (containing two filtered feeds) in many popular Web-based aggregators.

11.5.3
Other Tools for Filtering or Combining Feeds

Our favorite tool for manipulating feeds is unquestionably Yahoo! Pipes (http://pipes.yahoo.com/). Like most very powerful tools, though, its learning curve can be steep for beginners. If you're just getting your feet wet, you might want to try one of these tools:

- FEEDblendr – combining (http://feedblendr.com/)
- FEEDcombine – combining (http://www.feedcombine.co.uk/st/content/makefeed/)
- RSS Mix – combining (http://www.rssmixer.com/)
- FeedSifter – filtering (http://feedsifter.com/)
- FeedTwister – combining (http://www.feedtwister.com/)
- ReFilter – filter (http://re.rephrase.net/filter/)

11.6
Receiving RSS Items as Email

Sometimes you might find information that is available only via RSS, but decide that you'd like to receive this particular kind of informa-

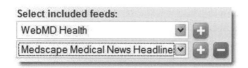

Fig. 11 Selecting feeds to combine in FeedRinse

tion via email instead of in your aggregator. When this is the case, there are a number of free services that make this easy to do.

To subscribe to an RSS feed via email using RSSFWD:

1. Navigate to RSSFWD (http://www.rssfwd.com/)
2. Paste the URL of the feed into the field at the top of the screen and click Submit
3. Enter the email address at which you'd like to receive emailed updates for this feed
4. Choose the frequency with which you'd like to receive emailed updates (one email for each new item, maximum of one email each day, etc.)
5. Click the Subscribe button

If RSSFWD doesn't meet your needs, you can try similar services like SendMeRSS (http://www.sendmerss.com/) or ZapTXT (http://zap-txt.com/). If you prefer, ZapTXT can also be set to send updates from an RSS feed to an instant messaging client or to your mobile phone/PDA.

11.7
Personalized Start Pages

If you really only want to subscribe to a small number of feeds, you might just skip the use of an aggregator and instead view your feeds on a personalized start page. Any RSS feed can be displayed as a module in most personalized start page services (see Chap. 12 for details).

11.8
Tips for Managing Your Feeds in Google Reader

An aggregator can allow you to review a massive amount of information, but some users find themselves overwhelmed quickly. Here are some tips specific to Google Reader to help keep that from happening to you:

- In the upper left corner of Google Reader (just below the "Add subscription" link) is a control for "Show" where the two options are "updated" and "all." Click "updated." This will mean that you will only ever see items that are new to you and you can't ever become confused about what you have already seen and what you haven't.
- Group related feeds together using Google Reader's labels. This will make it possible to review the items of multiple related feeds simultaneously.
- In the middle top of Google Reader, next to the name of the feed or folder, you'll see an option to view either all items from the feed or folder to view only the new items. Select only to view the new items.
- On the top right of Google Reader are tabs that allow you to select either Expanded view or List view. Select List view. List view will let you first see only the title of each feed item. This lets you skim items very quickly. You can expand and read the items that interest you, then click Mark all as read to mark all the items you skipped as read – and you'll be done with them forever.

There are more tips for using Google Reader and other aggregators efficiently in Chap. 14.

11.9
Moving Your Subscriptions to a Different Aggregator

If you decide that Google Reader isn't the right aggregator for you, you might consider switching to another aggregator but hesitate because it would be an awful lot of work to resubscribe to all of the feeds you're currently using. Fortunately, most aggregators have import and export functions that make your subscription list portable. When you export a list of feeds, it is usually as an OPML file. OPML stands for outline processor markup language, and it is yet another kind of XML-based document format,

but you don't really have to care. All you really have to know is that an OPML file contains all the details about the feeds you're subscribed to.

To export your feed list from Google Reader in an OPML file:

1. At the bottom left of Google Reader, click "Manage Subscriptions"
2. Click Import/Export
3. Click "Export your subscriptions as an OPML file"
4. Choose "Save to Disk" and save this OPML file to your computer somewhere you'll find it again easily. The Desktop would work well. The default name for this file will be "google-reader-subscriptions.xml"

Now, if you want to load this list of feeds in a different aggregator, just look for that aggregator's Import function and tell it to upload the OPML file you just saved to your Desktop.

Some aggregators will export an OPML file with the file extension ".xml" at the end of it, others will use ".opml" – any good aggregator should recognize what the file is, regardless of which extension it is using.

To import a feed list from another aggregator into Google Reader:

1. At the bottom left of Google Reader, click "Manage Subscriptions"
2. Click Import/Export
3. Where Google Reader says "Select an OPML file," browse to the OPML file you exported from another aggregator
4. Click Upload

Since OPML makes switching aggregators easy, don't be afraid to try new ones to see how you like them! Google has assembled a list of links with notes on how to export a list of feeds as an OPML file from various Web-based aggregators that may be helpful: http://www.google.com/support/reader/bin/answer.py?hl=en&answer=70572

11

11.10
Check in with Your Medical Librarian

Your medical library may have a lot of suggestions for RSS feeds you might want to utilize and may have RSS-based services that would be useful to you. For example, the University of Wisconsin-Madison Ebling Library for Health Sciences has a terrific RSS service available for its users (http://ebling.library.wisc.edu/rss/index.cfm) that organizes feeds for news and journals alphabetically or by subject and makes subscribing to them easy. The Harvey-Semester JournalBot (http://www.harvey-semester.de/news/journalbot) can help guide the physician toward the feeds that may most interest him/her (in either English or German).

Personalized Start Pages 12

you can customize them, create your own content, share your content, and generally manage your Web experience. It's possible to add any RSS feed to a personalized start page, so you can add the tables of contents for all your favorite medical journals and scan them in one page.

Most personalized start pages are also productivity tools. They offer notepads, to do lists, calendars, email access, bookmarks, and more. Netvibes and Pageflakes also connect with your accounts on many of the other Internet cool tools like Facebook (see Chap. 20), Delicious (see Chap. 18), and Flickr.

12.1
Personalized Start Pages

You already have a start page on your Web browser. Maybe it's your institution's Intranet page or maybe it's a search engine. Whatever your starting place on the Web is, can it deliver news, weather, email, instant messaging, journal tables of contents, and the rest of what you need and want on the Web in a single location? Personalized start pages can. They are your home away from home online.

There are several excellent personalized start page services available, all for free. The most popular are My Yahoo!, iGoogle, Netvibes, and Pageflakes. These tools are so useful because

12.2
My Yahoo! (http://my.yahoo.com)

My Yahoo! is the most popular of the personalized start pages. It serves as a portal not only to your Yahoo! services like email, but also to a wealth of news, tools, and other information.

To use My Yahoo! at multiple computers, you'll need a Yahoo! account. If you don't have a Yahoo! account, you can create one at https://edit.yahoo.com/registration. Yahoo! requires a substantial amount of personal information to create an account, however. If you choose not to use a Yahoo! account, you can create a My Yahoo! page for whatever computer you are using.

M. Rethlefsen et al., *Internet Cool Tools for Physicians*
© Springer-Verlag Berlin Heidelberg 2009

12

12.2.1
Setting Up My Yahoo!

The first time you go to the My Yahoo! page, you may be prompted to set up a My Yahoo! page in three steps or you may be prompted to click on "Personalize this page" to begin. At any time, clicking on the Personalize this page button is the way to add content, change the look and feel of your page, and change other options.

My Yahoo! is comprised of modules (sometimes called gadgets or widgets) with different types of content like local news stories, television listings, and weather. You can remove modules by clicking the X in title bar of the module you want to remove. Moving modules around on the page is as simple as dragging and dropping the module. One great feature is that by scrolling over a title of an article, a pop-up window will give a summary or abstract when available.

Search and browse for new modules in the Personalize this page area. Click on Add Modules to access the available modules. The categories are browseable, but the real power of My Yahoo! is in searching for modules. Unlike some other personalized home pages, whenever someone creates a new or unique My Yahoo! module based on an RSS feed (see Chap. 11 for more information on RSS feeds), it will be searchable. There are millions of My Yahoo! modules, including modules for hundreds of medical journals, PubMed searches, and many other good sources. Search for a keyword of your choice and click on the Add button next to the module listed. My Yahoo! displays a preview of the module before you commit to adding it.

You can also create your own My Yahoo! module with any RSS feed (see Chap. 11). From the Personalize this page area, choose Add RSS Feed. Just paste in the URL for the RSS feed and click on Add to create the custom module. Individual modules can also be customized by clicking on the gear icon in the title bar for any given module (Fig. 1).

12.2.2
Recommended Modules

Health and medically oriented modules include:

- Journal tables of contents (New England Journal of Medicine, JAMA, etc.)
- Health news (Washington Post Health News, Johns Hopkins Medicine Weekly Health News, NPR: Health & Science, etc.)
- Organizational and group news (Doctors without Borders, Student Doctor Network Forums, etc.)

Modules with helpful tools are also common:

- Currency converter
- Stock portfolios
- Calendar
- Bookmarks

To add these modules, search by keyword.

12.3
iGoogle (http://www.google.com/ig)

iGoogle is Google's version of the personalized start page. In place of the austere single search box and plain white background, you can morph your iGoogle start page into a colorful and useful tool for managing your information.

Though you can use iGoogle without creating a Google Account, to take advantage of iGoogle's transportability, you'll probably want an account. That way, you can access your iGoogle start page from any computer with Web access. If you don't create an account, your iGoogle settings will stay on a single computer.

12.3.1
Personalizing iGoogle

Once you've gone to the iGoogle page and created your account, what next? Now comes the fun part – personalizing the page. The first time you

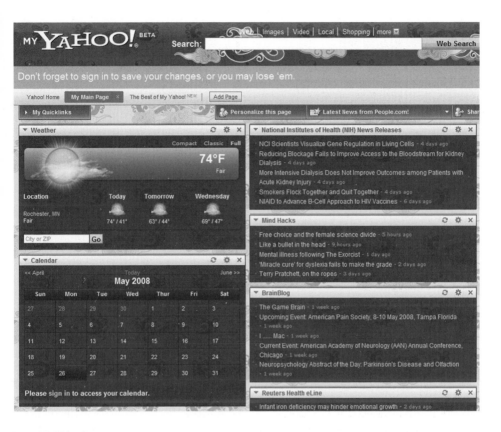

Fig. 1 My Yahoo!

go to iGoogle, you'll be prompted to select your interests and a theme (a background) for your iGoogle page. If you select one or more interests, iGoogle will populate itself with things it thinks you might like. You can also opt to skip this step and go to the basic default page.

iGoogle is made up of customizable gadgets. By default, iGoogle usually includes a clock and calendar gadget, a weather gadget customizable to your location, news, and other general gadgets. If you selected an interest or interests, iGoogle will create additional tabs with gadgets in that topic area. To remove gadgets, it's as easy as clicking on the X in the top right corner. You can also rearrange the gadgets on the page just by dragging the title of the gadget to a different spot or a different tab (Fig. 2).

To add content, click on Add Stuff. This takes you to the searchable Gadgets directory. Simply browse by category or search for a keyword to find new gadgets. If you find one you like, click on Add it Now.

Thousands of gadgets are available, ranging from stock quotations, games, calculators, sports scores, specialized search engines, and nearly everything you can imagine. There are lots of medically oriented gadgets as well, offering medical news, medical terminology dictionaries, consumer health Web site portals, grant information from the National Institutes of Health, and more.

A number of medical publishers and journals have created their own iGoogle gadgets with tables of contents, medical news, and medical images. These include:

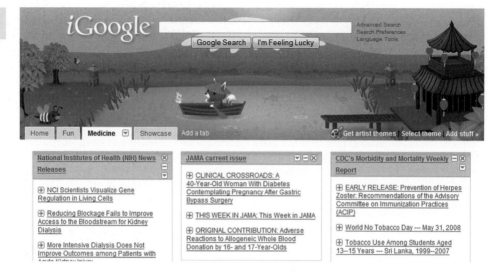

Fig. 2 iGoogle

- New England Journal of Medicine (tables of contents, image challenge, image of the week, popular articles, audio summaries)
- JAMA (tables of contents)
- BMJ (tables of contents, latest headlines, BMJ Clinical Evidence)
- Lancet (tables of contents, podcasts)

Try searching for your favorite medical journals – chances are, you'll find a gadget!

> If you add a news gadget or a medical journal gadget, look for the plus signs next to the article title. Clicking on the plus sign will often give you a summary or abstract of the article right in the gadget.

Many gadgets can be customized by selecting the arrow on the title bar. One particularly helpful customizable gadget is the Google News gadget. You can use the gadget to keep up to date on a particular type of news or a topic by entering a keyword of your choice. After adding the gadget, select the arrow and enter your choice of keyword or select one or more types of news, customize the number of news items to display, and even change the font used by the gadget.

What happens if your favorite medical journal doesn't have its own gadget? You can create one. All you need is an RSS feed (see Sect. 11.3 for information on finding RSS feeds). Find the link to Add Feed or Gadget located in the left-hand side of the gadget directory. Paste in the URL for your RSS feed, click on Add, and you've created a custom gadget.

> If you use Delicious (see Chap. 18 for more information on Delicious), numerous iGoogle gadgets exist to help you access or search your Delicious bookmarks.

12.3.2
Adding and Sharing Tabs

One of the best things about iGoogle is the tabs. You can create as few or as many tabs as you choose, allowing you to organize different types of information on different tabs. To create a tab, simply click on the Add a Tab link next to your existing tabs. Name the tab whatever you choose. If you would like iGoogle to find gadgets for you, leave the "I'm feeling lucky" box checked. iGoogle will try to identify gadgets related to whatever you named the tab. If you want to start with a blank slate, simply uncheck the box.

So, now you've created the perfect iGoogle page and have neatly organized all the information you need on one or more tabs. Perhaps your friends, family, or colleagues would benefit from the work you've put in, especially if you created a medical journal portal customized for your needs. Luckily, you can share any iGoogle tab with another iGoogle user. Just click on the arrow on the tab you want to share and enter an email address. It's also possible to pick and choose what gadgets in the tab to share at this step.

12.4
Netvibes (http://www.netvibes.com)

Netvibes is perhaps the most elegant of the personalized start pages. It is easy to use, highly customizable, and rich with content and productivity tools. To sign up for a Netvibes account, click on Sign In in the top right

corner of the Netvibes page. Netvibes opens a left sidebar with an option to Register now. Registration requires only an email address and password (Fig. 3).

In Netvibes, the modules or gadgets are called *widgets*. Like in My Yahoo! or iGoogle, you can add as many or as few widgets as you like. Widgets can be rearranged by dragging and dropping, removed by clicking the X on the title, and options changed through the down arrow in the title bar. To see the options for each widget, mouse over the title bar. In addition to the basic functions, there's also a refresh icon to refresh the data in any given widget. Widgets that have news articles or journal articles will often have pop-up summaries or abstracts when mousing over titles, much like in My Yahoo!.

To add new widgets, click on the Add content link in the top left corner. This will open a navigation bar on the left of the screen. Many popular widgets are accessible directly from this sidebar – look under Widgets. Alternately, browse through or search all the available widgets by selecting Browse content at the top of the sidebar. Over 100,000 widgets are availa-

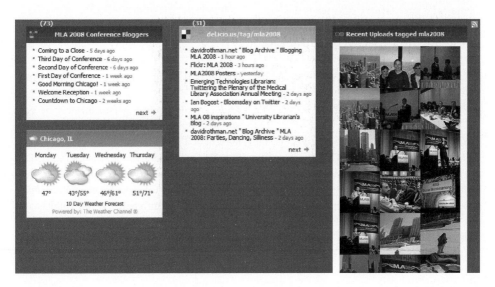

Fig. 3 Netvibes

12

ble in Netvibes, including a Facebook widget (see Chap. 20 for information about Facebook) and a Delicious widget (see Chap. 18).

Not as many medical journals are represented in Netvibes as in My Yahoo! or iGoogle, but you can easily create your own widgets from an RSS feed, a Web page, or any custom HTML code. To create a widget, click on Add content. To create a widget for an RSS feed, select Add a Feed from the top of the sidebar. Paste in the URL of the RSS feed of your choice to add it as a widget.

You don't need to have an RSS feed to create a widget in Netvibes. In fact, you can add any Web page you want in your Netvibes page. This is very useful for those Web pages without RSS feeds or that you visit regularly. To create a widget for a Web page, scroll down to the bottom of the sidebar and look for External widgets. In the External widgets menu, select Web Page, click on the edit button, and paste in the URL or Web address for the Web page of your choice. A miniature version of the Web page will be added to your Netvibes page.

> If you have an RSS reader or aggregator setup with your favorite RSS feeds, but you want to switch over to using Netvibes, you are in luck. You can import OPML files into Netvibes under the Add a Feed option. What's OPML? Check out Sect. 11.9 for more information. This is the fastest way to add content to your Netvibes page.

One of Netvibes' coolest features is the HTML widget. Using the HTML widget, you can paste in any HTML code you want and have it display in a Netvibes widget. What is that good for? There are almost limitless possibilities, both for those savvy at HTML and those with no knowledge of HTML – really. The best

use of this option is to create a widget with code that another Web site provides.

One Web site that provides this kind of code is YouTube (http://www.youtube.com). For each YouTube video, YouTube provides embed code that you can copy and paste into the Netvibes widget. This will put a YouTube video directly into your Netvibes page. You might want to include a medical procedure video, for example. YouTube is far from the only Web site providing this kind of option – look for widgets, embed code, and other codes on your favorite Web sites.

If you create a widget, you can share it with your colleagues. To share a widget, click on the arrow in the title bar. There are three options: sharing the widget via email, sharing via instant messaging, and sharing it via a blog or MySpace. The last option generates code that you can paste into a Web site, a blog sidebar, or anywhere you can add a widget.

> Netvibes has a version for the iPhone (http://iphone.netvibes.com). If you are an iPhone user, you can get all your RSS feeds, news, to do lists, Facebook access, and more – all through the Netvibes iPhone Web site.

12.5
Pageflakes (http://www.pageflakes.com)

Pageflakes is another personalized start page option. Pageflakes is as slick as Netvibes with the feel of a social network. Most like Netvibes, Pageflakes can help you access the news, RSS feeds, and productivity tools you need. The main difference is that the modules are called *Flakes*. The other main difference is the emphasis on community. You can create Pagecasts, or collections of Flakes, to share with others.

Your myopia progressed a lot ...

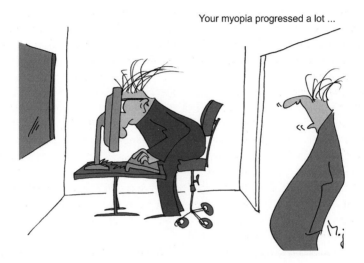

Podcasting and Vodcasting

13

Core Messages

> Podcasting is the delivery of an audio file via an RSS feed.

> Podcasts are available from a great number of useful and authoritative sources and can help you stay up to date on the go.

Podcatcher. Software for downloading the audio from podcast feeds

Podcasting is a method of distributing audio files via syndication feeds (RSS or Atom).

But that doesn't really clear anything up, does it?

13.1
What Is Podcasting?

Essential Podcasting Vocabulary

iPod. Apple, Inc.'s line of portable music players

MP3. A compressed file format that allows audio files

MP3 Player. A piece of software or portable device that allows the user to listen to an MP3 file

Podcast (noun). An RSS feed that delivers audio files

Podcast (verb). To make audio files available via RSS for distribution/syndication

Podcasting. A method of distributing a compressed audio file via an RSS feed

Podcaster. A person who creates and/or maintains podcasts

13.1.1
MP3s

When they first came out, CDs were pretty exciting for a lot of people. They allowed audio to be encoded digitally on round, plastic discs with fidelity that had audiophiles throughout the world impressed. As personal computers became more popular and people started working with their audio files on their computers, it became clear that the files taken directly from CDs had a problem: they took up a lot of space. This meant that audio files were slow to download or upload and not a whole lot of them could be carried around.

MP3s solved this problem. The MP3 file format could compress the data of an audio track and deliver the same song (at a level of audio quality not discernible to most users from a CD) in a file format as much as ten times smaller than the way it was recorded on a CD. Since these audio files were now much smaller, they

M. Rethlefsen et al., *Internet Cool Tools for Physicians*
© Springer-Verlag Berlin Heidelberg 2009

13

could quickly be uploaded or downloaded online and a massive number of tracks (songs, usually) could be stored very efficiently. Savvy manufacturers figured out that if they made devices that could play these compressed files, consumers could carry around huge music collections on small devices. Collectively, we can call these devices "MP3 players," but the most successful player is the iPod, manufactured by Apple, Inc.

13.1.2
MP3s Delivered via RSS

In Chap. 11, we discussed RSS feeds, which deliver just the content you want to your aggregator. A podcast is essentially an RSS feed wherein each item contains a link to a compressed audio file, usually an MP3.

There are audio files on my iPod that aren't MP3s! Do all podcasts deliver MP3 files, or can they deliver other kinds of compressed audio files?

There are related audio file types like AAC or MP2 which accomplish much the same thing as MP3s (compressing audio to smaller files for easier sharing). For the purpose of this chapter, you can read "compressed audio file" for every time we use "MP3," but MP3 is overwhelmingly the format of choice in podcasting – so we don't mind oversimplifying a bit on this point.

13.2
Receiving Podcasts

13.2.1
Receiving Podcasts in a Feed Aggregator

You don't need an iPod (or other brand of MP3 player) to subscribe to a podcast. You can subscribe to a podcast feed as you would any other feed. Depending on your choice of aggregator, you may be able to listen to the audio file in the aggregator itself or you may need to click on a link in your aggregator to download the audio file. An additional layer of usefulness can be achieved by using a podcatcher.

13.2.2
Receiving Podcasts in a Podcatcher

A podcatcher is a specialized kind of feed aggregator for subscribing to podcast feeds. A podcatcher will recognize the link to an audio file that is contained in each item of a podcast feed and download it. Some podcatchers just download the audio file and queue it up for the user to listen to later. Other podcatchers will download the file and copy it to the user's MP3 player whenever the MP3 player is plugged into the computer. That way, your MP3 player is loaded up with the latest audio files from your favorite sources every time you take it off its cradle. The best-known podcatcher is probably iTunes, but there are a number of options for Windows, Mac, and Linux operating systems.

Some Podcatchers to Try

These podcatcher applications are free and full of useful features:

- iTunes (Available for Windows or Mac): http://www.apple.com/itunes/download/ (note: you do not need an iPod to use iTunes)
- Juice (Available for Windows, Mac, or Linux): http://juicereceiver.sourceforge. net/index.php

One of these two choices should suffice for most, but for help choosing a podcatcher that will meet your specific needs, go to http://www.podcatchermatrix.org/

13.3
Listening to Podcasts

13.3.1
How Will I Listen to Podcasts If I Don't Have an iPod or Other MP3 Player?

If you use a Windows computer, these files will probably automatically open in Windows Media Player unless you have defined another audio player to open and play audio files. If you use a Mac, these files will automatically open in iTunes.

13.4
What Is Vodcasting?

A vodcast (sometimes called a vidcast, a videocast, or a video podcast) is just like an audio podcast except that instead of delivering a compressed audio file, it delivers a video file instead of an audio file.

13.5
Where Do I Find Podcasts?

Below are just tiny samplings of what's available from the podcasting world.

13.5.1
Medical Journals and Associations

- JAMA: http://jama.ama-assn.org/misc/audio-commentary.dtl
- The JAMA Report: http://thejamareport.blip.tv/rss
- The Lancet: http://www.thelancet.com/audio
- New England Journal of Medicine: http://content.nejm.org/misc/podcast.dtl

- Annals of Internal Medicine: http://www.annals.org/podcast/index.shtml
- Nature: http://www.nature.com/nature/podcast/index.html
- AAC Conversations with Experts: http://conversations.acc.org/
- Society of Critical Care Medicine: http://www.sccm.org/SCCM/Publications/iCritical+Care/

13.5.2
Government Agencies

- Agency for Health Research and Quality: http://www.healthcare411.ahrq.gov/
- U.S. Centers for Disease Control: http://www2a.cdc.gov/podcasts/
- U.S. Food and Drug Administration: http://www.fda.gov/CDER/drug/podcast/default.htm
- U.S. National Institutes of Health: http://www.nih.gov/news/radio/nihpodcast.htm
- U.S. National Library of Medicine: http://www.nlm.nih.gov/listserv/rss_podcasts.html

13.5.3
Patient Education

- The Cleveland Clinic: http://www.hopkinsmedicine.org/mediaII/Podcasts/podcasts.html
- The Mayo Clinic: http://www.mayoclinic.org/podcasts/

13.5.4
Medical Education

- Cleveland Clinic Medical Education Podcasts: http://www.clevelandclinicmeded.com/online/podcasts/
- Johns Hopkins: http://www.hopkinsmedicine.org/mediaII/Podcasts.html

13

13.5.5
Directories, Lists, and Services
for Healthcare Podcasts

- JournalJunkie: http://www.journaljunkie.
  com/

- Duke University Medical Center Library
  Podcast List: http://www.mclibrary.duke.edu/
  subject/podcasts
- LearnOutLoud: http://www.learnoutloud.com/
  Podcast-Directory/Education-and-Professional/
  Medical

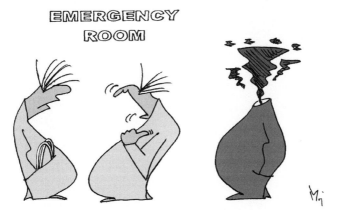

He was downloading his emails at a hotspot location ...

Organizing with RSS Readers

> RSS readers offer great ways for you to manage your information, whether by using folders and tags or by creating your own database of information.

> Use sharing features to send information to your friends and colleagues.

14.1
Why Organize?

Once you've started using RSS, it's pretty hard not to find it addictive. You may find that there is so much great information out there that you struggle to keep up. Though we can't stop people from producing information, we can offer you a few tips for keeping your RSS life under control. In the examples below, Google Reader is the RSS aggregator we'll talk about, but remember that other aggregators like Bloglines also have excellent features for organizing, managing, and sharing your RSS experience.

14.2
Google Reader Folders

The simplest way to keep Google Reader and your incoming feeds under control is to use folders. Your folders can be named anything you choose, but one of the best ways to assign feeds to folders is to think about your feeds in terms of priority. If you have one or two feeds that it is absolutely critical that you read everyday, assign those to a critical folder. If you have lots of feeds that you'll only read if you have time, assign them to a low-priority folder. Then, you can mark all the new items as read if you need to, without worrying too much about missing something important. You can also create folders with feeds for specific projects or on specific topics – whatever your preferred way to organize, you can do it with folders.

When you subscribe to a feed in Google Reader, you'll be given an option to add that feed to a folder. You can add it to one or more existing folders or create a new folder. If you are reorganizing your folders, go to the Subscriptions tab in Settings. You'll see a list of all the RSS feeds you've subscribed to, along with options to change folders. To add feeds en masse to a particular folder, check the boxes next to your selected RSS feeds and

M. Rethlefsen et al., *Internet Cool Tools for Physicians*
© Springer-Verlag Berlin Heidelberg 2009

use the More Actions menu to select the folder you wish. (In the More Actions menu, the folders are called *tags*, but it's the same thing in this case.)

14.3
Subscribe, Mark Read, and Search Later

Now that Google Reader has search functionality built right in, you can use it as more than your RSS reader. You can make Google Reader into your own personal database. Google Reader's search functionality lets you search all items, items in a particular folder or from a particular RSS feed, or in starred or shared items (see Sect. 14.4 for more information on starred and shared items).

This means that you can subscribe to feeds that you may not even need right now, but that you might want information from later. Google Reader will hold the contents of that feed for you until you need it. Simply put feeds you don't need to read right away in a particular folder or folders, mark all items as read, and search later at your leisure.

14.4
Starring and Sharing Items

If you want to read something later or want to mark an item, star it. Starred items are given their own folder and are searchable as well as browseable. The star is to the left of each post title.

Shared items are a little like starred items, insofar as you select particularly good posts, but unlike starring, which is a private method of marking items, sharing items enables you to create a clip blog that you can share with friends, family, or colleagues. Clip blogs are blogs you create without creating your own content (see Chap. 15 for more information on blogs). There are two ways to share items publicly: sharing individual items and sharing items with a particular folder or tag.

To share individual items, simply click on the Share icon at the bottom of each item. This will put the item into your shared items Web page. Your shared items Web page has a URL you can share along with an RSS feed.

You can also share items based on a public folder or tag. To set up a public tag, go into the Tags tab in Settings. Each tag (or folder name) that you have used is listed by default as private. Click on the Share icon to make your tag/folder public. Once you've made a tag/folder public, Google Reader provides a link to the Web page with your shared items that you can send to friends or colleagues.

One of the best things about sharing items by a public tag is that you can easily create several clip blogs for different groups of people. For instance, you could have a public tag for friends, a public tag for family, one for all your colleagues, and one for the colleagues with whom you're working on a particular project. You can customize the items you share with each group, and it is far more private than sharing items via using the Share icon (Fig. 1).

Why is using a public tag/folder more private? In late 2007, Google Reader introduced an intrusive new feature. If you have a Gmail or GTalk account (Google's email and instant messaging clients), if your contacts use Google Reader, your shared items will start appearing in their Google Reader account. This doesn't happen to items that are shared with public tags/folders. Newly introduced privacy measures allow you to control which contacts you share your items with and let you see who is sharing their items with you.

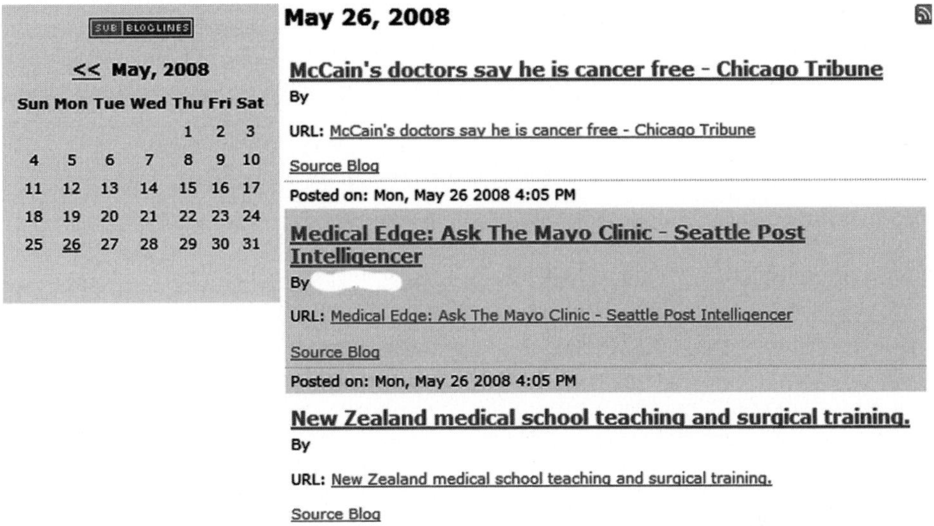

May 26, 2008

Fig. 1 A clip blog created using the Bloglines RSS reader. Similar functionality is available in Google Reader

14.5
Tags

Google Reader confusingly conflates folders and tags, so it's somewhat hard to distinguish which is which when. Basically, whole feeds are organized in folders on the left side of your reading pane. You'll see the folder icons that you can expand and contract to show or hide the feeds in your folders. However, the names of your folders are also called tags. Like any other tag (see Sect. 18.2 for more information on tags and tagging), it's just a keyword that you assign. Where the tag designation makes more sense is when you tag an individual item.

At the bottom of each item, you can edit the tags. Items in folders will already have tags attached, but you can delete these from individual items or add new tags. The only real rule is to separate multiple tags with commas. Remember that you can share items via a public tag.

Blogs

15

Core Messages

› "Blog" describes a kind of Web site, not a kind of content.

› Blogs allow anyone to produce and syndicate serially updated content at very low cost.

› Numerous sources exist to help you find the blogs of greatest interest/use to you.

15.1
What's a Blog?

You can hardly read a magazine or watch the news lately without hearing about blogs. Actors, musicians, and athletes have blogs. Cable news talking heads have blogs. Candidates for and occupiers of elected offices have blogs. Corporations and executives have blogs. That's all well and good…unless you're not sure what a blog is.

Most agree that the word "blog" is a blending of the words "Web log." A blog is a type of Web site made up of dated entries (called "posts") that are usually displayed in reverse chronological order with the most recent post at the top of the blog's main page. Each post can also be

reached at its own unique URL (address), usually called a "permalink" (for "permanent link"). Most blogs invite readers to leave comments, and each post has its own small discussion forum. Blogs are easy to create and maintain, requiring virtually no prior knowledge of Web markup languages. If you can write a letter in a word processor, you have the skills necessary to create and maintain a blog.

15.2
Why Are Blogs Such a Big Deal?

It used to be that to start publishing a newsletter, the aspiring publisher would need a minimum investment of resources to get it up off the ground. The skills and materials of production and distribution didn't come cheaply, after all – and the publisher couldn't hope to have a newsletter break even financially unless he could count on an interested audience that would be large enough to sustain it.

Blogs changed all that. Blogs can be created and maintained at sites like Google's Blogger (http://www.blogger.com/) or WordPress (http://www.wordpress.com/) at absolutely no cost. Blogs are easy to learn how to use and anyone can put together a professional-looking layout in no time. Even better than how blogs make production

M. Rethlefsen et al., *Internet Cool Tools for Physicians*
© Springer-Verlag Berlin Heidelberg 2009

15

Essential Blog Vocabulary

- **Archives** – Navigable list of previous posts, organized by date for easy browsing
- **Blog** (noun) – A particular type of Web site made up of dated posts in reverse chronological order. Usage: "Where did I hear about that study? On a blog by a Cleveland Clinic physician."
- Blog (verb) – When used as a verb, to blog is to update or maintain one's blog (noun). Usage: "That was an interesting differential – maybe I'll blog about it."
- Blogger – A person who contributes items (posts) to a blog. Usage: "Paul Levy is not just the President and CEO of Beth Israel Deaconess Hospital, he's also a blogger."
- **Archives** – Navigable list of previous posts, organized by date for easy browsing
- **Blog** (noun) – A particular type of Web site made up of dated posts in reverse chronological order. Usage: "Where did I hear about that study? On a blog by a Cleveland Clinic physician."
- Blog (verb) – When used as a verb, to blog is to update or maintain one's blog (noun). Usage: "That was an interesting differential – maybe I'll blog about it."
- Blogger – A person who contributes items (posts) to a blog. Usage: "Paul Levy is not just the President and CEO of Beth Israel Deaconess Hospital, he's also a blogger."
- Blogroll – A list of blogs, usually placed in a blog's sidebar. The presence of a blogroll usually implies that the blog's author reads and recommends the blogs in his/her blogroll.
- **Categories/tags** – Many blogging systems allow the blogger to assign one or more categories (or tags, depending on which blogging system is in use) to each blog post. This allows users to browse posts by topics indicated by those tags and provides additional structured data about each post that can make posts easier to find by those using blog search tools like technorati.com.

Essential Blog Vocabulary

- **Permalink** – A link to a particular blog post
- **Sidebar** – A blog frequently has one or more sidebars placed (sensibly enough) on the side of the blog's screen. Sidebars may contain search fields, links, blogrolls, navigation for browsing previous posts by date, categories or tags for browsing previous posts by topic.
- Splog – The word "splog" is a blend of "spam" and "blog," indicating a blog setup for dishonest marketing or search engine optimization purposes. The content of a splog is frequently taken without permission from the work of others. Splogs are frequently encountered when using general blog search engines, but a user can learn to recognize them pretty quickly.

inexpensive, they make distribution free, fast, and far reaching in that readers can subscribe to receive new posts via email or RSS feed (see Chap. 11 for more information on RSS).

With the barriers of expenses involved in production and distribution all but eliminated, anyone (or any group of people) can start publishing and stand a good chance at reaching a larger audience of those who share their specialized interests.

15.3
Why Read Blogs?

The best reason to follow a few good blogs is that they can be an excellent source of current awareness. The amount of new information that becomes available each day can be overwhelming, but following a handful of trusted blogging colleagues can make the daily avalanche of new information much more easily digestible. Some medical bloggers read all the health news and can distill it down to just the pertinent details of just the most important stories in a first-person, informal style that allows the reader to quickly follow up if his interest is peaked. Because blogs can be so incredibly specialized, there are at least a few excellent bloggers providing regular updates and useful commentary on new developments in virtually every specialty and subspecialty. Perhaps most importantly, blogs can be lots of fun and a way to network with colleagues.

15.4
How Do I Find Blogs That Will Interest Me?

15.4.1
Blog Search Engines

There are many search engines that specialize in searching the content of blogs, and some do it more successfully than others. The three general blog search engines we like best are Technorati (http://www.technorati.com/), Google Blog Search (http://blogsearch.google.com/), and Ask.com Blog Search (http://www.blogsearch.ask.com/). While these search engines can be useful, they cast a very wide net in attempting to index tens of millions of blogs, so it can sometimes be difficult to wade through the search results that will inevitably contain items from low-quality blogs or splogs (see sidebar).

15.4.2
Search MedWorm

Unlike Technorati, Google Blog Search, or Ask.com Blog Search, MedWorm (http://www.medworm.com) will allow you to limit a search just to medical blogs. Just below the search entry form are several square check boxes. Check the box for blogs and uncheck all the others, then perform your search (Fig. 1).

By using the tabs at the top of the page, MedWorm can sort your search results by relevance or by date (which is useful for seeing how some conversations may be distributed across several blogs over a period of time) or filter the posts displayed by what category of blog they came from (Fig. 2).

This specialized kind of granular searching allows the user to be very specific. For instance, if you wanted to see only the most recent posts from Family Medicine physicians about cardiologists, MedWorm can deliver exactly that (http://www.medworm.com/rss/search.php?qu=cardiologist*&r=Any&blogs=on&ftc=85a&o=d).

15.4.3
Browse MedWorm's Blog Directory

MedWorm maintains a Blog Directory (http://www.medworm.com/rss/blogs.php) that will allow you to browse medical blogs by category.

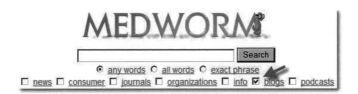

Fig. 1 Searching MedWorm for blog posts

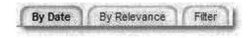

Fig. 2 MedWorm's filtering tabs allow filtering by date or relevance

15

Interested in emergency medicine blogs? Click on the link for that category and review snippets of the several most recent posts from blogs in that category. If you'd prefer just to see a list of blogs that make up this category, click the Sources tab and review the list of blogs with notes on when each was last updated (blogs that go a long time without updates are rarely particularly good).

15.4.4
Browse the Healthcare100

The Healthcare 100 (http://www.edrugsearch. com/edsblog/healthcare100/) is an attempt to rank the "top" healthcare blogs by adding together various methods of estimating popularity. There are two important things to remember about sites like the Healthcare100. First, that the measurements it uses can be wildly inaccurate and varying. Second, many of the Web sites seem to want to use "popular" as a substitute for "authoritative" or "high quality." With that said, we can note that there is definitely a lot of overlap between medical blog popularity and quality (the most popular blogs often really are among the best) and that browsing the list of the top 100 blogs on the Healthcare100 is a great way to find out what others who share your interests seem to enjoy.

15.4.5
Review the Blogrolls of Blogs You Know You Like

Once you've found a blog or two that you really enjoy, check their sidebars and look for their blogrolls. A blogroll is a list of blogs placed in the sidebar by a blog's author, and usually implies that the author enjoys, reads, and recommends these blogs. If you enjoy Kevin, M.D. (http://www.kevinmd.com/blog/), take a few minutes to review Kevin's "Blogs

of Note" and see what blogs he thinks are worth checking out.

Some Blogs We Like

- **Kevin, M.D.** (http://www.kevinmd.com/) – Dr. Kevin Pho, an internist in New Hampshire, reads a massive amount of healthcare news and blogs everyday and shares the highlights of what he finds on his blog. If you don't have time to follow all of the news that might be of interest to a physician, it might well be worth subscribing to Dr. Pho's blog and let him follow it for you.
- **Clinical Cases and Images – Blog** (http://casesblog.blogspot.com/) – This consistently interesting blog written by Dr. Ves Dimov features case histories, medical news, images, and useful practical technology tips.
- **Running a Hospital** (http://runningahospital.blogspot.com/) – Paul Levy, President and CEO of Beth Israel Deaconess Medical Center in Boston, gained a large readership very quickly with his candor and eagerness to post quality data on his blog about his hospital. He also invites stakeholders (patients, physicians, allied health professionals) to use his blog to comment on and ask questions about Beth Israel Deaconess.
- **Polite Dissent** (http://politedissent. com/) – Dr. Scott Morrison is a physician in Family Practice with a love for television and comic books. He frequently offers critiques of medicine being portrayed with something less than realism in his favorite pop cultural products. The detailed notes on made-up drugs from comics in Scott's Comic Book Drug Reference (http://politedissent.com/cbdr.html) are entertaining, but his biggest claim to fame is through

his medical reviews of each episode of House, MD (http://www.politedissent.com/house_pd.html). Dr. Morrison's skillful and entertaining deconstruction of each episode of the Fox Network's medical drama has earned so much attention that he now does some consulting for medical dramas on the side.

15.5
Tips for New Bloggers

- Start by signing up for a free blog at Google's Blogger (http://www.blogger.com/) or at WordPress (http://www.wordpress.com/). Both services will keep your blog on their servers and both have easy-to-learn interfaces. If you decide later that you'd like even more control over your blog or want to host it on your own server or hosting service, you can do so very inexpensively.
- Immediately set up your blog's feed to go through Feedburner (http://www.feedburner.com/). This will allow you to track the number of subscribers to your blog, to easily create a form through which readers can subscribe to your blog, and to move your blog to another platform or address without making your readers have to follow you or resubscribe.
- Read lots of other blogs. You can't carve out your own little corner of the blogosphere unless you know the terrain.
- Be social and interact with other bloggers. Leave comments on other blogs, comment on things that you read on other blogs and link to other blogs.
- Post regularly. You don't have to post daily, but you'll disappoint and lose readers if you go too long without updates. Try to post at least weekly.
- Know how to stay out of trouble. For some guidelines on legal matters relating to blogging see:
  - Electronic Frontier Foundation: Legal Guide for Bloggers (http://w2.eff.org/bloggers/lg/)
  - 12 Important U.S. Laws Every Blogger Needs to Know (http://www.avivadirectory.com/blogger-law/)

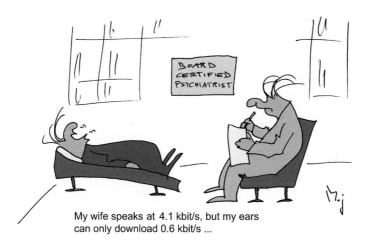

My wife speaks at 4.1 kbit/s, but my ears
can only download 0.6 kbit/s ...

Core Messages

› Wikis are Web sites that allow collaborative development of content.

› Some wikis are more reliable than others and the physician can learn to judge reliability.

› There are a number of health information wikis of potential use to physicians (and to which physicians may wish to contribute).

16.1
What's a Wiki?

A wiki is a kind of Web site that allows multiple people to collaboratively write or edit content, even with little or no knowledge of programming or Web markup languages. The name for this kind of site comes from a Hawaiian word meaning "fast." Wikis are a big deal for two basic reasons.

First, wikis make it easy to build rich, complex sites with almost no specialized knowledge of Web markup languages because they either use a WYSIWYG ("What You See Is What You Get") interface that is no more difficult than a word processor or use a simple, easy-to-learn "wiki markup."

Second (and more importantly), wikis allow any number of people to develop content collaboratively. Imagine having a Web page that you and any number of people to whom you want to grant access can share information, build documents, and edit each other's work.

The idea is easier to grasp if we look at a specific example: Wikipedia.

16.2
Wikipedia: The World's Most Famous Wiki

The most famous application of a wiki is undoubtedly Wikipedia (http://www.wikipedia.org/), an online encyclopedia which anyone with an Internet connection can edit. The policy of allowing anyone to contribute has helped Wikipedia achieve an extraordinary breadth unparalleled in any other work of reference. At the time of this writing, the English-language version of Wikipedia contains more than 2.3 million articles.

Go to any article in Wikipedia and you'll find a series of tabs across the top of the page. The article tab shows the current version of the article. The discussion tab provides a forum where contributors can discuss various aspects

16

of the article. The edit this page tab gives the user access to make any changes to the content or appearance of the page and have those changes made by clicking the Save Page button at the bottom of the screen. The history tab keeps a detailed record of what changes were made and by whom. If a recent revision is deemed incorrect, the page can be "rolled back" to a previous version in the history. If users care a lot about a particular topic, they can subscribe to an RSS feed (see Chap. 11 for more information about RSS) for the changes made in that article to be alerted when any new changes are made.

Wikipedia's policy of allowing anyone to edit most pages isn't, however, the only model. The administrator(s) of a wiki can choose to allow participation to whatever extent best suits their purposes. The Citizendium (http://en.citizendium. org/) seeks to create a more trustworthy online encyclopedia through "gentle expert oversight." Contributors must use their own real names (as opposed to a user name or alias) and must apply to be approved as an author or editor (http://en. citizendium.org/wiki/Special:RequestAccount) by the site's administrators.

There is a tremendous amount of detailed health information in Wikipedia, but the authors of this book caution against placing too much faith on what you find there.

16.3
How Are Wikis Being Used in Healthcare?

General medical reference resources like UpTo Date are popular and many clinicians find them useful, but they are very expensive and frequently unavailable to clinicians working outside a well-funded academic setting. A number of clinicians in various parts of the world have realized that useful medical reference resources could be inexpensively created through collaboration and free wiki software. Among many others are these standout examples.

16.3.1
AskDrWiki

AskDrWiki (http://www.askdrwiki.com/) is a nonprofit effort managed by Kenneth Civello MD, MPH; Brian Jefferson MD; Shane Bailey MD; and Mike McWilliams MD – all of the Cleveland Clinic. AskDrWiki has adopted a number of editorial policies (http://www.doctor-wiki.net/2007/05/editorial-policy-published. html) to ensure that the information found there is trustworthy and of high quality. AskDrWiki requires that contributors contact the administrators to identify themselves and their credentials before they are approved for access to submit or edit articles, and all contributions they make are associated with their real names. Articles are regularly reviewed by section editors. AskDrWiki's costs are paid exclusively by donations, it does not accept advertising, and all contributors must disclose potential conflicts of interest.

16.3.2
Ganfyd

Its name derived from the phrase "Get Note From Your Doctor," Ganfyd (http://www.gan-fyd.org/) is a collaboration of physicians and medical students (mostly in Australia and the United Kingdom) which also requires those who wish to contribute to provide evidence of credentials (http://register.ganfyd.org/register. php) before being allowed to write or edit information on the wiki.

16.3.3
WikiDoc

Founded by C. Michael Gibson, MS, MD and with an editorial board populated by physicians from several prestigious WikiDoc (http://www. wikidoc.org/) has not yet obtained nonprofit status, but it is funded by donations only. WikiDoc will allow anyone to register and add or edit information, but users must apply and be approved by the site's administrators to become a section "editor-in-chief."

16.3.4
WikiBooks

Run by the nonprofit Wikimedia Foundation (which also runs Wikipedia), there are a number of WikiBooks on a variety of health topics (http://en.wikibooks.org/wiki/Medicine), and there are Wikiversity "schools" for Pharmacy (http://en.wikiversity.org/wiki/School:Pharmacy) and for Medicine (http://en.wikiversity.org/wiki/School:Medicine).

> Finding More Health Information Wikis
>
> http://davidrothman.net/list-of-medical-wikis (English language)
> http://medecine.2.0.free.fr/doku.php/wikis_medicaux (French language)

16.3.5
Specialty Wikis

There are a number of wikis dedicated to particular specialties. A handful of these are dedicated to radiology, including Radiopaedia (http://www.radiopaedia.com), the Radiology Wiki (http://www.radiologywiki.org/), and RadsWiki (http://www.radswiki.net/). WikiEcho (http://www.wikiecho.com/) is a resource for echocardiography and WikiSurgery (http://www.wikisurgery.com/) is an encyclopedia of surgery.

16.3.6
Medical Book Publisher Wikis

Any doubt that commercial publishers of medical texts find user-created wiki medical reference

tools a threat to their business model was removed in November 2007 when Elsevier (a major player in medical publishing) unveiled WiserWiki (http://www.wiserwiki.com/). Elsevier cleverly got their medical wiki off to a great start by "seeding" it with the contents of a book they publish, Textbook of Primary Care Medicine (3rd Edition) by John Noble. It should be noted that, not surprisingly for a resource run by a for-profit publisher, WiserWiki contains advertisements and does serve Elsevier's for-profit interests.

16.3.7
MacSurgWiki

McMaster University's Department of Surgery maintains its residency manual on the MacSurg-Wiki (http://wiki.mcmastersurgery.com/). The advantage of using a wiki to maintain such a manual is that updating the manual is quick, easy, and simple – and could be done by anyone authorized to make changes to it.

16.3.8
WikiHealthCare

The Joint Commission has created WikiHealth-Care (http://wikihealthcare.jointcommission.org/) "to enable and encourage discussion and collaboration among all users for the purpose of improving healthcare quality." Anyone who registers can write or edit content on WikiHealthCare.

16.4
Evaluating and Using Wikis

Physicians frequently (and rightly) ask if it is wise to trust information found on wikis. In the opinion of this book's authors, Wikipedia can be sensibly used in about the same circumstances you'd use Encyclopedia Britannica. It is a good place to get

16

a quick, basic overview of a topic and perhaps pointers toward more detailed and authoritative information. An unwise use of Wikipedia (or almost any other wiki) for health information would be to stop there and not move on to other more detailed and authoritative resources.

The quality of information found on wikis varies greatly – but there are factors that can help the physician estimate how trustworthy the information on a particular health information wiki might be. The most reliable health information wikis will:

- Check the credentials of contributors before allowing them to add/alter information
- Require contributors to use their own real names (not aliases)
- Post and execute detailed editorial policies which include a review process to make sure that multiple clinicians check over information posted
- Post the names and contact information for the wiki's administrators

- Have a revision history that reveals an active community of individuals who are reading and tweaking the content to improve it

16.5
Creating a New Wiki

If you're considering using a wiki to meet a professional need, consider visiting WikiMatrix (http://www.wikimatrix.org/). The WikiMatrix Choice Wizard can help you narrow down the many options by asking you a series of questions about your specific needs and preferences.

If you're not intent on hosting the wiki yourself or if you just want to try playing with one, we recommend signing up for a free account at PBWiki (http://pbwiki.com/) or at WetPaint (http://www.wetpaint.com/). Both of these services provide free hosting, a powerful set of tools, and useful options.

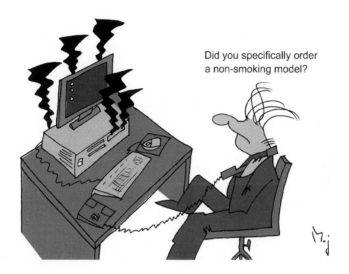

Collaboration Tools

17

Core Messages

> Stop getting buried by dozens of versions of documents when collaborating with groups on editing. Instead, create and edit your documents online in a single version.

> Online word processing, spreadsheet, and presentation tools mean never needing a standalone office software package, plus make sharing easy.

> Calendaring, project management tools, and online meeting tools make sharing and collaboration even easier.

17.1
Working Together: Online

You may be perfectly happy with your current desktop software for word processing, creating spreadsheets, calendaring, and presentations, but as wonderful as these desktop programs are, they are cumbersome when working with other people on projects. Email inboxes can quickly fill up with attachments, making it difficult to determine the most recent version of any document. Even when sharing a single copy of a document on a network drive, editing can quickly spiral out of control as multiple people edit a document.

New online office tools can help put a stop to the chaos. For instance, using an online word processor like Google Docs or Zoho Writer lets you keep a single copy of a document, see exactly who made what changes when, collaborate with others on the document in real time, and compare multiple versions of documents. You can even revert to an older version if necessary. Online office tools don't have all the bells and whistles that the desktop versions do, but they are perfect for working on documents with others, and even better, they are usually free.

Office applications aren't the only kinds of tools being pushed online. Where there is a need for collaboration, entrepreneurs have found a way to create an online tool to help. Project management tools and Web conferencing applications are two other types of tool that can help you collaborate.

17.2
Word Processing

Several excellent online word processing tools are available for your use. Which one you use depends on your personal preference, the features you want, and, most importantly, which ones

M. Rethlefsen et al., *Internet Cool Tools for Physicians*
© Springer-Verlag Berlin Heidelberg 2009

17

you can convince your colleagues to use. Luckily, most of these applications look and feel much like Microsoft Word or other standard desktop word processors, so they are easy to learn once you get used to the idea of working online. We'll cover two options, Google Docs and Zoho Writer, as examples.

17.2.1
Available Online Word Processors

- Google Docs (http://docs.google.com)
- Zoho Writer (http://writer.zoho.com)
- Microsoft Office Live (http://www.officelive.com/)
- ThinkFree (http://www.thinkfree.com)
- OpenGoo (http://www.opengoo.org/)
- Versionate (http://www.versionate.com/)

17.2.2
Using Google Docsv

If you already have a Google Account, you can log into Google Docs at http://docs.google.com. If you don't have a Google Account, you'll need to create one to use the service. You can create a document by uploading a document you're already working on (use the Upload button on the main Google Docs page) or start with a new blank document.

> You can also upload existing documents to Google Docs via email. Look in the Upload area for the special email address.

Once you've logged in and started a new document, Google Docs operates much like a regular word processor. Simply start typing. Most formatting options such as fonts, text size, and text format are available. Using the Document Settings in the File menu, you can even double-space your document. Standard editing tools like find and replace, undo and redo, and word count are also features. Using the Insert menu, you can add comments, images, links, tables, special characters, headers and footers, and page breaks to your document. There's a built-in spell check, too (Fig. 1).

To see how your document has changed, go to the File menu and select Revision history. All revisions are numbered, and you can check in the boxes next to two or more revisions to see exactly how your document has changed. You can also look at or revert to an older version of your document. If more than one person is collaborating on a document, you'll be able to see who made specific changes.

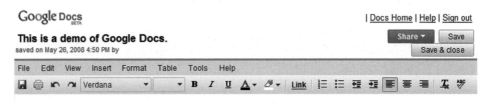

Fig. 1 A Google Docs word processing document

To collaborate with another person on a document, use the Share button to send an invitation to that person. You can add people as collaborators (they can edit the document) or as viewers (they can see the document, but can't edit it). Those people you invite to share your documents will require a Google Account to edit the document, though they'll be able to view it even without one. If you invite a collaborator who doesn't have a Google Account, they'll be given an opportunity to create one.

If more than one person is editing a given Google Docs file at the same time, Google Docs will notify you who the other person is. You'll see their changes as well as any you make in real time. You don't need to wait for someone to log out before editing.

If you're collaborating on a document, you can also use an RSS feed to keep up to date with the changes that are being made. From the Share button's Share with Others page, click on "View RSS feed of document changes." You can subscribe to the RSS feed, though the feeds may not work in all readers.

One of the special features of Google Docs is the readability check. When you perform a word count from the Tools menu, in addition to the number of words and approximate number of pages in your document, you'll also see three readability scores: the Flesch Reading Ease score, the Flesch–Kincaid Grade Level, and the Automated Readability Index.

Once you've finished your document, or if you need to share it offline, there are several options. First of all, Google Docs will export as HTML, Word (doc format), OpenOffice, PDF, RTF, and plain text. Depending on which format you choose to export your document as, you may lose some formatting or functionality. You can also publish your document on the Web using the Publish tab. You can choose to publish the document on your blog or just as a Web page on Google Docs.

The main Google Docs page lists your documents, spreadsheets, and presentations. By default, these are organized by date last updated. You can organize your files into folders, star specific documents for easy retrieval, hide items, and delete items. To create new folders, use the New menu and select Folder. To move items to a folder, you can drag the item to a folder or use the Move To button. Google Docs automatically lists shared documents by individual shared with below the folders list (Fig. 2).

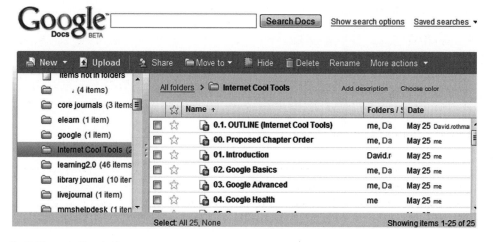

Fig. 2 The main Google Docs page

17

Google Docs now has an offline component. To use Google Docs offline, first install Google Gears (http://gears.google.com/). Google Gears also lets Google Reader users access their RSS feeds offline (see Chaps. 11 and 14 for more information on Google Reader).

17.2.3
Using Zoho Writer

Using Zoho Writer requires a Zoho account. To get started, go to http://www.zoho.com and click on Sign Up. You'll need to set up a username and password and have a valid email address. Once you're registered and logged in, you're ready to start using any of Zoho's free products, all listed on the main Zoho page (http://www.zoho.com). Zoho Writer (http://writer.zoho.com) is Zoho's word processing program.

To create a new document, click on the New button or import an existing document. Many of the features in Zoho Writer are the same as Google Docs as well as other word processing programs. Using the toolbar across the top of

your document, you can format text, check spelling, add images, insert tables, add comments, and much more. All the formatting options and features are available right from the toolbar, not hidden in menus (Fig. 3).

You can add an existing document to your Zoho account via email attachment. Look in the Import menu for the special email address to use.

Like Google Docs, Zoho Writer keeps track of your revision history, so you can compare different versions or revert to an older one. To access your revision history, click on History. Versions are numbered and are accessible from a drop-down menu. If you want to get back to your live document, click on Edit.

You can invite others to collaborate with you on Zoho Writer documents using the Share link. By default, Zoho Writer will invite your collaborators to view your documents only. If you want to grant full editing privileges, make sure to select the read/write option when you invite

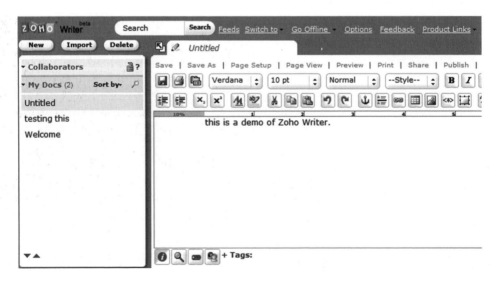

Fig. 3 Zoho Writer

someone. People who don't have a Zoho account will only be able to view shared documents until they register for a Zoho account.

As with Google Docs, more than one person can edit a Zoho Writer document at one time. You'll see the changes on your document in real time as others edit.

Zoho Writer's printing and page setup features are substantially more powerful than Google Docs' current offerings. Using the Page Setup link, it's possible to edit margins, line spacing, fonts, and header and footer information. You can also set margins by dragging them in the main editing window. The PageView link provides a quick look at what your document will look like in print, complete with page numbers.

If you have multiple files open at once, Zoho Writer will open them in tabs in the same window. This makes navigating between multiple documents a little easier. Simply click the X on the tab to close a particular file. You'll also always see your files listed on the left side of the screen.

You can add tags to help organize your documents at the bottom of the screen. Click on Tags to add one or more tags to a document. If you want to organize your documents into folders, click on a particular tag and select Add as Folder.

17.3
Spreadsheets

Most Web office suites also have a spreadsheet application. Though the spreadsheet functionality is not nearly as powerful in an online tool as it is in a standard desktop spreadsheet application like Microsoft Excel, the online spreadsheet tools are adding more functionality every day. Below, we'll look at two applications, Google Docs and Zoho Sheet, but many others are available.

17.3.1
Spreadsheet Tools

- Google Docs (http://docs.google.com)
- Zoho Sheet (http://sheet.zoho.com)
- Microsoft Office Live (http://www.officelive.com/)
- ThinkFree (http://www.thinkfree.com)
- OpenGoo (http://www.opengoo.org/)
- Versionate (http://www.versionate.com/)

17.3.2
Google Docs Basics

Using Google Docs spreadsheets is very similar to using Google Docs word processing (see Sect. 17.2.2), but with traditional spreadsheet functionality. This functionality includes autofill tools, sorting, formulas, creating rules, formatting cells and text, hiding and unhiding rows and columns, and chart and graph creation. A couple of cool features that make Google Docs spreadsheets unique are worth paying extra attention to, though.

17.3.3
Chatting with Collaborators

As in the documents part of Google Docs, you can share spreadsheets and collaborate in real time. An added benefit for spreadsheets users is the chat functionality built right into any shared spreadsheet. If you and a colleague are editing the same spreadsheet at the same time, you can send messages back and forth in real time (Fig. 4).

17.3.4
Creating Live Surveys

You can also gather information through a form--a spreadsheet designed to collect live data from other people. It's basically a simple survey tool.

17

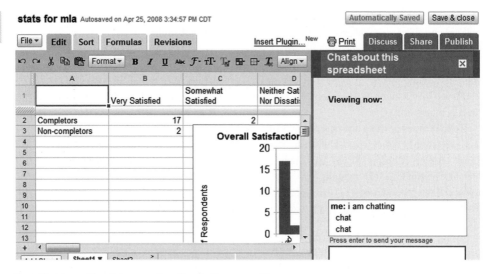

Fig. 4 Chatting with collaborators in a Google Docs spreadsheet

To create a form, select Form from the New menu. You can create questions with multiple choice (including radio buttons, check boxes, and drop-down choices) or free text answers (Fig. 5). Once you've entered in all your questions, you can invite participants to fill out your form or survey. The participants can respond to the form in their email or online. Once they've responded, your spreadsheet will start populating itself with the responses.

If you have an iGoogle personalized home page (see Sect. 12.3), you can create a gadget that shows your form responses. When you create a form, you'll receive an email with the link to the iGoogle gadget. Once you add it to iGoogle, you'll get live updates on how many people responded to your survey as well as a link to the results.

1.3.5
Special Functions That Automate Content

Though many of the special functions and formulas are in the English-language version of Google Docs, the functions and tools Google has created are very impressive and worth knowing about.

The first type of function is to automatically retrieve live-updating Google Finance information. You can create up to 250 Google Finance formulas to automatically retrieve price and volume for ticker symbols per spreadsheet. For more information, see Google Docs Help documentation at http://documents.google.com/support/spreadsheets/bin/answer.py?answer=54198 & topic=13320.

GoogleLookup functions enable you to try to pull facts into your spreadsheet from the Web. For example, you can create formulas to pull in:

- Country-, state-, and city-specific information like population
- Biographical or factual information on baseball players, actors, musicians, politicians, or U.S. presidents
- Chemical compounds or elements data
- Information on stars and planets
- Company data

For more information on using Google Lookup, see http://documents.google.com/support/

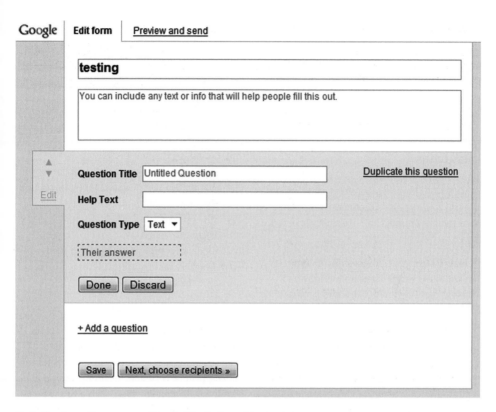

Fig. 5 Creating a live survey or form in Google Spreadsheets

spreadsheets/bin/answer.py?answer=54199& topic=13320.

In Microsoft Excel, you can use autofill to easily generate lists of numbers or fill cells with identical textual content. In Google Docs, you can use the autofill function to do the same tasks, but you can do even more with autofill. Using the power of Google Sets, a tool that predicts similar concepts based on one or more words, you can autofill your spreadsheet with lists based on a single word.

For example, if you were looking for information on medical device manufacturers, you could start by typing in Medtronic. Then, use autofill to find other medical device manufacturers by holding down the Control key (PC) or ALT key (Mac) and dragging the autofill. Instantly, your spreadsheet will list other similar manufac-

turers. This saves you some mental time (no more thinking of all the medical device manufacturers, for example) and a lot of typing.

To see these special functions in action, check out Google's short video on the topic on YouTube (http://www.youtube.com/watch?v=jVjwKm DLrIE).

17.3.6
Zoho Sheet

If you don't need the special automated content or survey functionality of Google Docs spreadsheet, Zoho Sheet (http://sheet.zoho.com) is a good alternative. It looks more like a traditional desktop spreadsheet program, and offers most

17

of the functionality you'd expect from a spreadsheet tool. Using Zoho Sheet requires a Zoho account and offers many of the same benefits as Zoho Writer does for word processing (see Sect. 17.2.3).

17.4
Presentations

As with word processing and spreadsheet applications, you can also create and collaborate on presentations online. Here are a couple of places to try:

- Google Docs (http://docs.google.com)
- Zoho Show (http://show.zoho.com)
- ThinkFree (http://www.thinkfree.com)

Embed a small version of your Google Docs presentation into your blog or Web site. Use the Publish tab to make your presentation public, and then copy and paste the code for the mini presentation into your blog or Web site. Visitors will be able to browse through your presentation directly on your site.

Want to share your presentations without needing to collaborate on them with others? You can use Web tools like Slideshare.net to upload your presentations and embed presentations on your blog or Web site. Using Slideshare.net, you'll also be able to receive comments from presentation viewers.

17.5
Calendars

Google Calendar (http://calendar.google.com) is one of many online calendaring tools. With Google Calendar, you can create multiple calendars. For each calendar that you create, you can make it completely public, make only the free/busy information public, share the calendar with designated individuals, or keep it private. You could create a calendar for friends, one for family, one for your practice schedule, or one for the conference that you'll be attending – or better yet, you could create all four. Each can be shared with whomever you choose at whatever level of permissions you select: read/write access, read-only access, or free/busy read-only access.

Physicians who want a free scheduling tool that patients can use to make appointments can use Google Calendar or another online calendaring tool. You could encourage patients to use an online calendar shared with you to keep track of their medical conditions. There are many uses for online calendaring applications – as many as you can think of.

One of the best features of Google Calendar is a new feature that enables syncing between Google Calendar and Microsoft Outlook. If you're tied to a Microsoft Outlook calendar but want the convenience of online access and individual-specific calendar sharing permissions, try Google Calendar Sync. For more information on installing this tool on your computer, see http://www.google.com/support/calendar/bin/answer.py?answer=89955.

The Clinical Cases and Images blog has collected lots of great examples of physicians and patients using Google Calendar. See http://casesblog.blogspot.com/2006/04/google-calendar-for-doctors-help.html for more tips and suggestions.

17.6
Project Management

For working on large projects, whether a clinical trial, a research project, or any other complicated project, project management software can be critical to success. Several online tools exist to help you with your projects, the most popular of which is Basecamp (http://www.basecamphq.com).

Basecamp and other online project management tools generally allow users to create one project at a time for free; beyond one project, most tools will charge a monthly or yearly fee for access.

What can you expect from a project management tool like Basecamp? Basecamp offers a number of features, some of which may not be accessible in a free version. Here's an overview of features you might see, based on Basecamp's features:

- Unlimited users per project for collaboration with large groups
- To do lists where to dos can be assigned to project members
- Messages/blogs for centralized project discussions
- Milestones to mark important due dates for project components
- Assignment of responsibility for to dos and milestones to members
- File sharing
- Chat tools for instant communication
- Project activity feeds to keep up with what's new
- Online document creation and sharing (similar to Google Docs)

Other project management tools include Zoho Projects (http://projects.zoho.com) and goplan (http://www.goplan.info).

17.7
Online Meetings

When you collaborate with people in disparate locations or even just in offices across the street, it's often easier to get online and meet instead of trying to schedule a video conference. Several online tools can help you set up spontaneous or planned online meetings for free. Most of these tools let you share your desktop with the other attendees so you can demonstrate Web tools, display word documents, or show off the features

in your electronic medical record system. With a few of them, you can even audio or video chat with other attendees.

17.7.1
Twiddla (http://www.twiddla.com/)

Twiddla is a new player in the online meeting market. Calling itself a team whiteboard, Twiddla lets you share Web sites, graphics, and photos and mark them up. You can add text notes to the whiteboard as well as draw or add shapes. When you're in a Twiddla meeting, you can use the audio chat feature to start talking to any attendees who have a microphone and speakers.

To start a Twiddla meeting, go to http://www.twiddla.com, click on Start a New Meeting, and invite your meeting participants via email.

17.7.2
Zoho Meeting (http://meeting.zoho.com)

Zoho Meeting is a desktop sharing application. It requires the presenter (the person controlling the computer) to have a Zoho account and a PC, but it will share more than a single application at a time. You can use Zoho Meeting to set up planned and scheduled meetings or to create spontaneous meetings. Zoho Meeting will send participants an email with a link to join the meeting. It's also possible to embed a meeting into a Web page for other viewers to watch.

Presenters can turn control of their desktop over to a meeting attendee, which makes it perfect for demonstrating software, troubleshooting, and collaboration. If you have a Skype account (http://www.skype.com), you can use audio with Zoho Meeting, though if you do not, there is a chat tool for instant messaging communication. If you want to add audio communication to your meeting without having a Skype account, you'll need to set up a separate phone conference.

17

17.7.3
Elluminate vRoom (http://www.elluminate. com/vroom/)

With vRoom, up to three people can conduct a free meeting online. Unlike Zoho Meeting and Twiddla, both of which have relatively few hoops to jump through to start a meeting, vRoom requires you to fill out a rather lengthy form before using the product. vRoom has more features than Twiddla or Zoho Meeting, however. With vRoom, you can share your desktop, browse the Web, chat over audio, use Web cams for virtual face-to-face communication, and much more.

Social Bookmarking

Core Messages

> Organize and access your bookmarks online using social bookmarking tools.
> Share bookmarks with colleagues, friends, and strangers who are interested in the same topics you are.
> Use tags or keywords to organize your bookmarks in a way that you'll be able to find them again – forget the folders.
> Use academic social bookmarking tools to share citations and references with your colleagues.

If you switch between computers frequently, but don't want to lose your special browser settings and bookmarks, try using Mozilla Firefox Portable Edition (http://portableapps. com/apps/internet/firefox_portable), a version of Firefox you carry around on a USB drive. An additional benefit for those sharing computers is that your browser history is private because you take it with you.

18.1
What Is Social Bookmarking?

In the past, to keep track of stuff you've seen on the Web, you had one option: using your Web browser's built-in bookmark function. Whether you used Internet Explorer, Netscape, or Firefox, the built-in bookmarking tool has its own problems. Even with the very best organizational skills, everyone's browser bookmarks tend to devolve into lengthy lists of disorganized, outdated content. Even worse, your bookmarks are tied to a single computer. If you tend to switch between computers, your bookmarks can get lost.

Social bookmarking is different. Social bookmarking tools offer two main benefits over regular bookmarking tools: organization and portability. For starters, social bookmarking tools are Web based. You can access them from any computer connected to the Internet, irregardless of what computer you used to bookmark them. Secondly, social bookmarking tools improve organization with tagging.

18.2
What Is Tagging?

Tagging is simply choosing a few keywords to describe a particular bookmark. In each social bookmarking tool, when you bookmark something, you can add keywords (called *tags*) to the

M. Rethlefsen et al., *Internet Cool Tools for Physicians*
© Springer-Verlag Berlin Heidelberg 2009

18

bookmark. Tagging helps you find your bookmarks again.

> Another bookmarking tool you can try is Google Bookmarks. Though Google Bookmarks don't offer the same social experience or organizational power that social bookmarking tools can give you, you will be able to access your bookmarks from any computer. It's a good choice for people who may only want a few bookmarks.

18.3
The Social in Social Bookmarking

Social bookmarking has one more major component that makes it so powerful – the social part of social bookmarking. What's so interesting about social bookmarking is that when you bookmark something, everyone can see it. This may seem like an invasion of privacy, and in part, it is. You are hidden behind the anonymity of a username of your choice, however, and in most of the social bookmarking tools, you can choose to make some or all of your bookmarks private.

Once you've experienced using a social bookmarking tool, you're going to want to have those bookmarks public. Many features depend upon the public connections you can make in these tools, particularly finding like-minded people who bookmark the same types of content you do.

18.4
Delicious (http://www.delicious.com)

Delicious is the classic social bookmarking tool. Owned by Yahoo!, Delicious has been around since 2003 and now boasts over two million registered users. To set up an account, go to http://Delicious/register. Registering requires you to create a username and password and have a valid email address. Once you've created an account, you'll install buttons in your browser (Internet Explorer, Firefox, Opera, and Safari only).

Once you have your buttons installed, you can start bookmarking. To bookmark something in Delicious, you can either click on your browser's new Tag button or post using http://delicious.com/save. Delicious will prefill the Web address and title of the Web page you are bookmarking for you, though you can edit either. The posting page is where you add tags, or keywords, to categorize your post (Fig. 1).

Tags are there to help you find your resources again, so the only real rule of tagging is to pick words or tags that make sense to you. Tags can be generic, like medicine or food, or directive, like toread or toblog. The more bookmarks you tag, the better you'll understand what tags work best for you.

> Until July 31, 2008, Delicious was known as del.icio.us. Delicious updated its spelling to make it easier for everyone to type and use. You will see Delicious and del.icio.us used interchangeably on the Web. Most tools for using Delicious will use the old name, and most hardcore Delicious fans will likewise refer to del.icio.us. With the name change came significant changes to the user interface as well. Many online tutorials and tip sheets will be for the old interface. Delicious itself is still as useful as ever.

18.5
Connecting with Others in Delicious

For every bookmark that's entered into Delicious, you can see who else bookmarked it by clicking on the number to the right of each bookmark. Each tag is also clickable, so you can see all of your bookmarks with a certain tag, or everyone's bookmarks with that tag. Exploring the network of bookmarkers is one of the best reasons to use Delicious. You can browse through tags, users, and bookmarked resources easily, and hopefully discover new and exciting Web content.

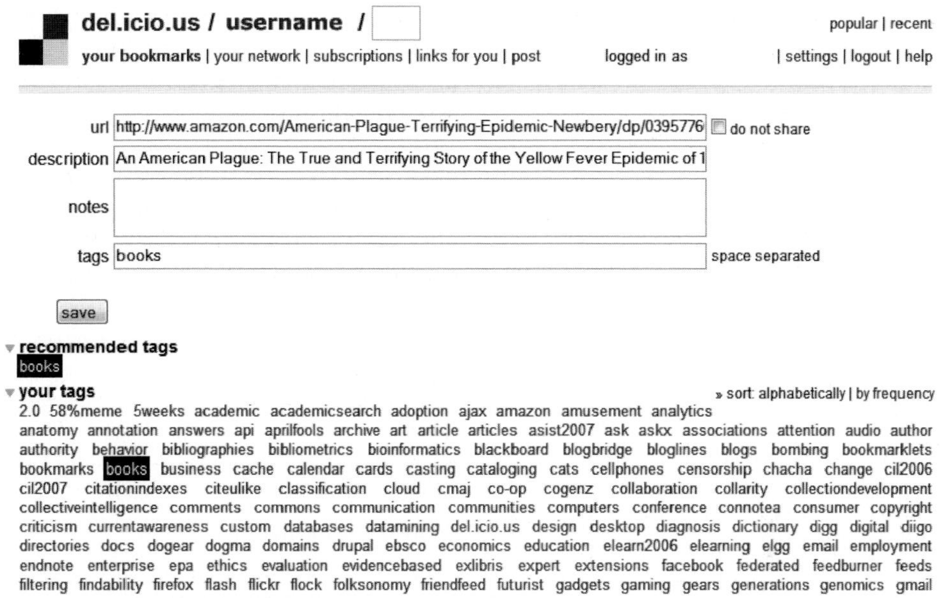

del.icio.us / username / ⬚

your bookmarks | your network | subscriptions | links for you | post   logged in as | settings | logout | help

url	http://www.amazon.com/American-Plague-Terrifying-Epidemic-Newbery/dp/0395776	☐ do not share
description	An American Plague: The True and Terrifying Story of the Yellow Fever Epidemic of 1	
notes		
tags	books	space separated

[save]

▼ **recommended tags**
[books]

▼ **your tags**   » sort: alphabetically | by frequency
2.0 58%meme 5weeks academic academicsearch adoption ajax amazon amusement analytics anatomy annotation answers api aprilfools archive art article articles asist2007 ask askx associations attention audio author authority behavior bibliographies bibliometrics bioinformatics blackboard blogbridge bloglines blogs bombing bookmarklets bookmarks [books] business cache calendar cards casting cataloging cats cellphones censorship chacha change cil2006 cil2007 citationindexes citeulike classification cloud cmaj co-op cogenz collaboration collarity collectiondevelopment collectiveintelligence comments commons communication communities computers conference connotea consumer copyright criticism currentawareness custom databases datamining del.icio.us design desktop diagnosis dictionary digg digital diigo directories docs dogear dogma domains drupal ebsco economics education elearn2006 elearning elgg email employment endnote enterprise epa ethics evaluation evidencebased exlibris expert extensions facebook federated feedburner feeds filtering findability firefox flash flickr flock folksonomy friendfeed futurist gadgets gaming gears generations genomics gmail

Fig. 1 Bookmarking a Web page in Delicious. The keywords on the bottom are tags that can be selected to describe the bookmark, or new tags can be added

If you find a particular Delicious user who seems to bookmark a lot of content you like, you can add them to your Network. Delicious, each user can subs cribe to any number of other users' bookmarks using the Network feature. When you add a person to your Delicious Network, whenever that person bookmarks something publicly, it shows up in your Network Page. You can use this feature to find new content or keep up to date with what your friends are up to. Just click on "Add to my Network" and either subscribe to the RSS feed for your network or just check your network page at your convenience.

Each Delicious user also has an Inbox. Links in your Inbox are ones that other people have bookmarked and thought you would like. To send links to another Delicious user, it's necessary to use a special tag – the for: tag. When you are tagging a bookmark and want to send it to another Delicious user, just add for:user (where user is the Delicious username) as another tag. The link will get sent to the other user's Inbox. Whenever a new link is bookmarked for a user with the for: tag, the user's inbox link will be bold and will list the number of new items.

Since it's possible to selectively make certain bookmarks private, you can also send another user a private link and message using the for: tag. Even better, if you've added a user to your network, you can easily send links to that person by clicking on their for: tag that automatically appears in your posting form.

18.6
More Delicious Goodies

18.6.1
New Firefox Extension (Firefox 1.5 or Higher Required)

Firefox users who want a little more Delicious power built into their browser can install the new Firefox extension (http://delicious.com/help/installff). The extension integrates your Delicious bookmarks into a Firefox sidebar. It also provides improved searching and organizational features.

18.6.2
Play Tagger

For music buffs and anyone using MP3 files, Play Tagger is a helpful tool. Any time you bookmark an MP3 file in Delicious, the Play Tagger lets you play it directly from Delicious. You can also get a Play Tagger bookmarklet (http://delicious.com/help/playtagger) to instantly add Play Tagger functionality to any Web page with MP3s.

18.6.3
Tools for Bloggers

One of the best things about Delicious is its flexibility – you can take your data with you, whether as an RSS feed, downloading all your bookmarks, or, if you are a developer, using the Delicious API or JSON feeds. Luckily, for the nondevelopers amongst us, Delicious provides some easy tools especially to help bloggers show off their Delicious accounts. With a simple cut and paste, bloggers can add a link roll (an updating list of your new bookmarks), a tag roll (a colorful "cloud" of all of your tags), and a network badge. The network badge displays the number of your fans (people who've put you in their network) as well as a quick link for blog readers to add you to their Delicious network. The tools for bloggers are available in the settings once you've logged into your account.

18.6.4
More Cool Delicious Tools

Delicious lists even more neat tools at http://delicious.com/help/thirdpartytools. These include link checkers to check for dead links in your Delicious bookmarks, alternate interfaces, and even visualization tools.

18.7
Managing Journal Articles and References Socially

After Delicious hit the scene, academics quickly saw the potential for using social bookmarking to manage and share journal articles. There are a few tools furnishing this kind of social reference managing – CiteULike, BibSonomy, and Complore are a few – but the main one focused on science and medicine is Connotea.

18.8
What Is Connotea?

Connotea (http://www.connotea.org) is a social bookmarking tool geared toward the scientist and clinician. Created and operated by the Nature Publishing Group, it is a tool that goes one step beyond generic social bookmarking tools to manage your journal article and book collections. What makes Connotea special is its ability to recognize journal articles, preprints, and books, to create group collections, and to facilitate collaboration and communication between scholars and researchers. With one click, you can add an online article to your Connotea library.

Connotea captures the bibliographic information (journal title, page numbers, etc.) for each article you bookmark, unlike a typical social bookmarking tool. That makes it much easier to refind articles you're interested in, as well as for creating bibliographies for grants or other publications. If you use EndNote or another bibliographic management software tool, you can import your citations directly into Connotea. Citations can also be exported back out. Connotea is compatible with many different online journal publishers and databases, including PubMed, BioMed Central, Nature, Science, Wiley Interscience, and Amazon. You can also include general bookmarks in your Connotea library, not just articles and books.

18.8.1
Using Connotea

As with Delicious, to use Connotea, you'll first need to register for an account, at http://www.connotea.org/register. Once you've registered, you'll install a Add to Connotea bookmarklet or button in your browser (Internet Explorer, Firefox, and Safari instructions are provided by Connotea).

After you've installed the bookmarklet, you're ready to start bookmarking articles in Connotea. From PubMed or while viewing an article on a publisher's Web site, simply click the Add to Connotea button to pop up a form where you can add your tags and notes to the citation information Connotea captures for you. You can use multiword tags in Connotea – just put quotation marks around any phrase (Fig. 2).

Connotea provides video tutorials and other help resources at http://www.connotea.org/guide.

You can also add citations to Connotea using the Add form (http://www.connotea.org/add). Though you can fill out this whole form by hand should you choose, you can also use a shortcut and add citations by DOI number or by PMID. DOI (digital object identifier) numbers are assigned to electronic journal articles by publishers to give each article a static identifier. DOI numbers are usually two sets of numbers and letters divided by a slash (e.g., 10.1038/nature06842). You'll often find them on print copies of articles, so if you're reading a print copy of an article, you'll be able to bookmark it in Connotea easily by entering doi: followed by the DOI number in the Bookmark URL field.

The PMID number is the PubMed identifier, a unique number assigned to each PubMed record. To add PubMed citations to Connotea, just type pmid: followed by the PMID in the Bookmark URL field. Unlike bookmarking the DOI, which bookmarks the article at the journal's Web site, bookmarking the PMID links to the PubMed record for the article.

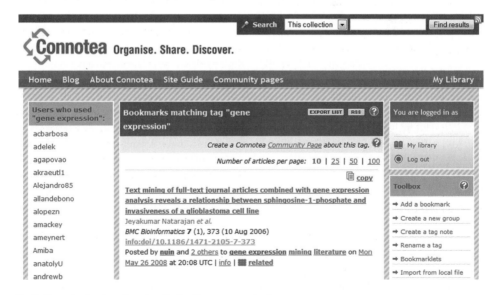

Fig. 2 Connotea bookmarks using the tag "gene expression"

18

18.8.2
Connecting with Other Physicians and Researchers

Connotea's social features aren't quite as impressive as Delicious' network capabilities, but there are a few built-in features making it easy to share references with colleagues. For every bookmark that's entered into Connotea, you can see who else bookmarked it by clicking on the "X people" link below the bookmark. Each tag is also clickable, so you can see everyone's bookmarks with any given tag. Exploring the network of bookmarkers is one of the best reasons to use Connotea. You can browse through tags, users, and bookmarked resources easily, and hopefully discover new and exciting Web content.

After you start bookmarking in Connotea, you'll also see a list of related users listed on the right side of your library. If you find a particular Connotea user who seems to bookmark a lot of content you like, you can subscribe to an RSS feed of all their new links or to a particular one of their tags.

Using the Connotea Toolbox on the right side of your Connotea library, you'll be able to create groups. Groups are public or private collections of Connotea links shared between two or more people. For instance, if the members of your practice wanted to collaborate together on a research project, you could use a group to have everyone assemble the resources they think are important. If you join a group, be warned that all of your links will show up in the group's page; there's not currently a way to designate particular links to send, either to a group or to an individual.

18.8.3
More Connotea Cool Tools

Connotea's users have created dozens of tools to help you make the most of Connotea, the majority of which require Firefox and the Greasemonkey extension. You can browse through these tools on Connotea's Community Pages (http://www.connotea.org/wiki/ConnoteaTools).

One of the tools is called Entity Describer (http://www.connotea.org/wiki/EntityDescriber), a pair of Greasemonkey scripts that help you tag articles in Connotea using a controlled vocabulary like MeSH (medical subject headings). Though a benefit of social bookmarking is coming up with your own tags, if you are working in a group or want to make sure that your tags are meaningful to others, the Entity Describer tool can help you find appropriate and standardized tags.

18.9
Other Social Bookmarking Options for Physicians

For now, Delicious, Connotea, and a few other established social bookmarking tools are the best bet for physicians. On the horizon, however, are social bookmarking tools designed solely for physicians. It's possible that these tools may become popular in the future, though none will ever have the power the sheer size and popularity Delicious commands.

PeerClip (http://www.peerclip.com) is one of a new breed of population-specific social bookmarking tools, this one geared just to physicians, nurse practitioners, and physician assistants. Right now, the site is in beta and can't verify your credentials just yet, but the plan is to run each member through a verification system to make sure that the community is exclusive. Other than its exclusivity, its only real difference from Delicious is that it doesn't work as well (Fig. 3).

CiteMD (http://citemd.com) is another social bookmarking tool geared toward physicians. CiteMD uses member voting to rank posts in addition to acting as a social bookmarking tool.

DissectMedicine (http://www.dissectmedicine.com/) is another social news tool. It's another Nature Publishing Group product, this one designed to present news headlines of interest to physicians. Users can vote on news stories, and the most heavily promoted articles make the main DissectMedicine page.

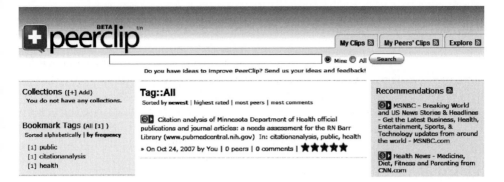

Fig. 3 Physician-only social bookmarking tool PeerClip

This is the latest office fitness exercise:
turn your screen upside down for an hour a day ...

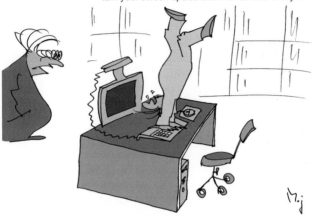

19 Keeping Notes

highlight and annotate text on the Web, and share your notes and annotations. Some of these tools are socially oriented – such as Diigo, Fleck, and SharedCopy. Some of these tools can be used to share with others, but are designed more for personal organization and use – such as Evernote, Zotero, and Google Notebook. Whichever the tool, it can help you organize and manage your information and research conveniently.

Core Messages

› For the times when it will take more than just a bookmark to keep your information organized, try social annotation or notebook tools to store, annotate, highlight, and organize your information.

› Share your information with colleagues, friends, and groups.

› Keep your references, your Web content, and your life organized with Web tools.

19.1
Keeping Notes

With social bookmarking tools, you can easily keep track of Web sites you've visited and share those sites with friends and colleagues. Social bookmarking sites like Delicious and social reference management sites like Connotea (see Chap. 18) are perfect for simple organization and sharing of Web sites. There comes a time, though, when what you really want is a little more power – the power to mark up the Web.

In this section, we'll go over a few different types of tool that all help you jot down notes,

19.2
Social Annotation Tools

The social annotation tools are like a combination of a social bookmarking tool, a highlighter, and sticky notes. Like with social bookmarking tools, saved links, highlights, and sticky notes are shareable, either with the entire community using the tool, a specified group of users, or just with one or more people to whom you send a link. Some tools even capture copies of each Web page you annotate and allow full-text searching of that content. Of course, your collection of links, highlights, and annotations are available wherever you have a Web connection.

Several of these tools also allow you to create Web tours, or a collection of annotated and highlighted Web pages in a specific sequence. Web tours can be used to demonstrate or comment

M. Rethlefsen et al., *Internet Cool Tools for Physicians*
© Springer-Verlag Berlin Heidelberg 2009

19

upon Web sites, show a particular set of resources to colleagues, or even to send an annotated collection of consumer health links to a patient.

With any social annotation tool, you won't get quite the same size of user community as you would at Delicious, for example, but the social aspect is not really diminished. This is because the power of social annotation tools is in sharing specific annotations via email or direct links, or in creating groups. Groups allow multiple people, perhaps a group working on a specific project, to highlight and annotate Web pages and share those annotations just with their group.

19.2.1
Diigo (http://www.diigo.com)

One of the most impressive social annotation tools is Diigo. Diigo has all the features you'd expect from a social annotation tool, plus a few extras. It is the most social of the social annotation tools, emphasizing community, friends, groups, and personalized recommendations. You can also post to Diigo and Delicious simultaneously using Diigo's bookmarking tools. To get started with Diigo, go to http://www.diigo.com/, sign-up and register.

Once you've created an account, you'll be prompted to install the Diigo Toolbar or the Diigolet. Installing the Diigo Toolbar is recommended because it offers far more features than the Diigolet. Most importantly, if you install the Diigo Toolbar, you can accomplish nearly all Diigo functions through the context (or right-hand click) menu – even if the Diigo Toolbar is hidden. The Diigo Toolbar also offers a sidebar for easy navigation of your bookmarks, sticky notes, and annotations. The Diigo Toolbar is available for Firefox, Internet Explorer, and Flock browsers.

The Diigolet is a lightweight version of the Diigo Toolbar that works like a bookmark let. It's recommended for users who may only use Diigo irregularly or for those who don't want to

install a toolbar. The Diigolet is the only option for Safari or Opera browser users as well, though it is also available for Firefox, Internet Explorer, and Flock.

If adding another toolbar to an already full browser doesn't thrill you, it's okay. The Diigo Toolbar can be customized to your liking, whether you want it smaller, merged with another toolbar, or completely hidden. As long as it's installed, you'll still get the right-click context menu. For tips on customizing the Diigo Toolbar, see http://blog.diigo.com/2008/03/27/tip-of-the-day-how-to-customize-diigo-toolbar/.

19.2.2
Using Diigo

Once the Diigo Toolbar is installed, you're ready to start bookmarking, highlighting, and annotating the Web. Let's say that you suspect a patient has malaria and you are doing some research on the Web to determine the best course of action to take for treatment. You've done a PubMed search to find some research articles, and you've also found some good Web resources using a search engine. How can you use Diigo to help organize the information you've found?

To merely bookmark any particular resource in Diigo, you have two options. First, you can use the One-Click Bookmark tool in the Diigo Toolbar. This bookmarks the resource on your Diigo page in one single step if you don't have the time or inclination to add tags or a description to your bookmark. To add tags or a description, or to make your bookmark private, or to share it with friends or a group, you would instead select the Bookmark option in the toolbar or by using the right-click context menu. All bookmarks show up on your Diigo bookmark page along with the tags and descriptions you add.

If you like the One-Click bookmarking option, you can change the default tags Diigo will add to your bookmarks under the Bookmark pull-down menu. By default, Diigo also marks One-Click bookmarks as unread, so you can figure out which ones to go back and read or annotate later.

That option is not much different from a regular social bookmarking tool, however. What makes Diigo special are its extra tools. Let's say that you found a particularly interesting journal article that you want to bookmark. Once you bookmark it, Diigo will save a copy of that Web page for you. That means that even if that Web page should disappear from the Web, you'll still have a copy saved on Diigo. To access the saved version of any Web page, click on the Cached link for the appropriate bookmark in your Diigo bookmark list.

The article you've found is pretty long, so you want to mark the parts most important to you. You can use the highlighting tool to highlight as much or as little text as you want. After you've highlighted a portion of text, you might want to add a sticky note (a floating comment) to that highlight. To do that, mouse over the highlighted text and select Add sticky note. Sticky notes can contain a large amount of text and can be made private or public (shared with the Diigo community).

It's also an option to add a sticky note anywhere in the article without highlighting any text. Either use the Comment pull-down menu to choose Add a floating sticky note to this page or right-click and select the same option. Floating sticky notes can be added anywhere on the page, and as many or as few as you want can be added (Fig. 1). If you just want to comment on the whole Web page, click on the Comment link in the toolbar.

All highlights and annotations (sticky notes and comments) are saved by Diigo. They'll be available both from the Web page itself the next time you visit and from your Diigo Web page. Click on the Expand link next to any of your Diigo bookmarks to view your annotations and highlights (Fig. 2).

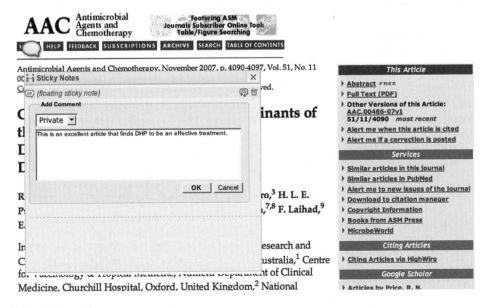

Fig. 1 A Diigo sticky note

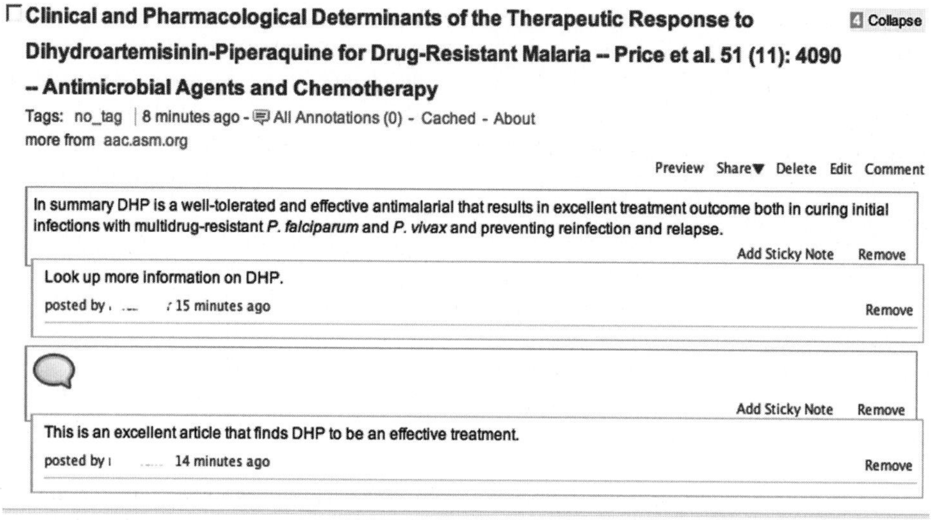

19

┌ **Clinical and Pharmacological Determinants of the Therapeutic Response to**   ▢ Collapse

Dihydroartemisinin-Piperaquine for Drug-Resistant Malaria -- Price et al. 51 (11): 4090

-- Antimicrobial Agents and Chemotherapy

Tags: no_tag │ 8 minutes ago - 🖘 All Annotations (0) - Cached - About
more from aac.asm.org

                                                                                 Preview   Share▼   Delete   Edit   Comment

┌───┐
│ In summary DHP is a well-tolerated and effective antimalarial that results in excellent treatment outcome both in curing initial │
│ infections with multidrug-resistant *P. falciparum* and *P. vivax* and preventing reinfection and relapse. │
│   Add Sticky Note   Remove │
├───┤
│ Look up more information on DHP. │
│ posted by , ._.. ⁏ 15 minutes ago   Remove │
├───┤
│ ◯   │
│   Add Sticky Note   Remove │
├───┤
│ This is an excellent article that finds DHP to be an effective treatment. │
│ posted by ⎹   ._... 14 minutes ago   Remove │
└───┘

Fig. 2 A personal Diigo account listing highlights and annotations for a bookmarked item

Let's say that your patient with malaria had lots of questions about the disease, and you want to share some high-quality Web resources with him. You can create a WebSlides slide show and email the link. Any WebSlides show you want to share will be publicly viewable, though, so be careful.

To create a WebSlides show, first create a list by selecting Create a new list from the Add to List drop-down menu. Once you've named the list, go back to your list of bookmarks and check the boxes next to the bookmarks/annotations you'd like to share. Then use the pull-down Add to List menu to select which list you want to add your selected bookmarks to. Once your list is created and populated, you can click on WebSlides icon to open your list as a slide show. An option within the WebSlides presentation allows you to email the WebSlides link to anyone you choose.

**19.2.3
Social Diigo**

If you are working with colleagues on a research project or just on collecting good Web links, Diigo has a nice Groups feature that allows collaboration and sharing with one or more others.

To create a group, go to http://groups.diigo.com/create. The Groups creation form asks for a Group name, a URL keyword that will create your group's unique Web address, and a number of questions about privacy. Your group can be public or private to view, search, or join. Once those options are filled in, Diigo prompts the group creator to invite other users to the group by email.

Other social aspects of Diigo are similar to those found in Delicious or other social bookmarking tools, but Diigo makes them a little easier. For example, instead of randomly stumbling across users whose bookmarks you might be interested in, Diigo lets you search for friends or colleagues by email address. The Find Your Friends option will harvest your contact list in your email, if you choose, or you can search by individual email addresses.

You can also join public Groups, send messages to "friends" (anyone in your Diigo network is also called a friend), or find friends based on interests once you have enough bookmarks in the system. Diigo even features users so you can browse and find additional friends. You can send bookmarks to friends, just like the for: option in Delicious. To share a bookmark, look for the Share link in the bookmark. Choose Send To to share with one or more friends.

You can also get a copy of the URL for any Web page you annotate. From the Share link, select Get Annotated Link. This link can be sent to anyone you would like via email, instant messaging, or of course as a link in a Web page or blog. You can also send a link using the Toolbar's Send menu. Options to send links to Diigo friends, Facebook, and Twitter are available.

Bloggers can also use Diigo to create blog posts based on bookmarks, annotations, and highlights. Simply annotate and highlight as usual. Then, select To Blog from the Send To menu. The blog post will automatically include a link to the original page plus the full text of any highlights and annotations. Bloggers using any of the major blogging services including WordPress, TypePad, and Blogger amongst others can set up a connection to their blog (Fig. 3).

19.2.4
Other Social Annotation Services

Diigo is not the only social annotation service available. Other cool tools to try out are:

- Trailfire (http://trailfire.com)
- SharedCopy (http://sharedcopy.com/)
- Clipmarks (http://www.clipmarks.com/)
- Fleck (http://www.fleck.com/)

19.3
Personal Organization Tools

The tools discussed below are a combination of tools that can be used to share and tools that are really designed for single person access. All, however, are considerably less social than the social annotation tools discussed above. For

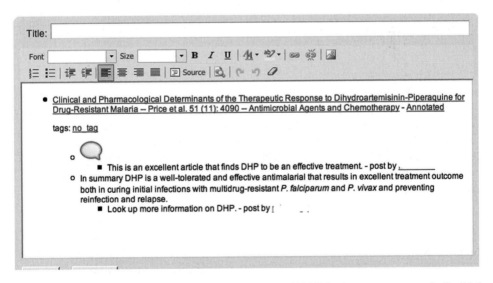

Fig. 3 Bloggers can use Diigo to create blog posts. Sticky notes and highlighted content are automatically added to a blog post about a bookmarked item

19

some purposes, such as research, creating a quick list of Web sites, or personal organization, these tools offer better alternatives or completely new tools.

19.3.1
Zotero

Zotero is a browser-based tool designed to help researchers. Firefox 2.0 or higher or Flock is required – Zotero is not compatible with Internet Explorer. With Zotero, you can easily capture copies of Web pages and PDF documents, tag these copies for easy organization and retrieval, annotate pages, and capture citation information that can be used to create bibliographies in Word and OpenOffice or as standalone bibliographies. Zotero is designed to replace EndNote or other bibliographic management software. Though it's primarily designed for humanities scholars, Zotero is nearly as useful for scientists and physicians.

19.3.2
Using Zotero

To use Zotero, you must be using Firefox 2.0 or higher or Flock as your browser. You can down-

load the Zotero add-on from the Zotero homepage (http://www.zotero.org/). Once you have the Zotero add-on installed, you are ready to start capturing and organizing your information.

Unlike Diigo or most annotation tools, Zotero does not live on the Web. You won't be able to access your Zotero information through a Web site or from a different computer. This is a major drawback of using Zotero currently, though Web access and social features are under active development.

> Zotero provides many video tutorials on using Zotero. Check them out at http://www.zotero.org/documentation/screencast_tutorials.

The Zotero add-on puts a Zotero icon in the bottom bar of the browser window. Clicking on this icon will open your Zotero library at any time. The Zotero library is a three-paned window offering access to all saved citations and copies of Web pages and PDF files. For each captured citation, you can add notes, attachments (such as Word documents, images, or PDF files), tags to help organize your collection, and links to related citations (Fig. 4).

To capture citations, click on the icon in the address bar of your browser. The icon will

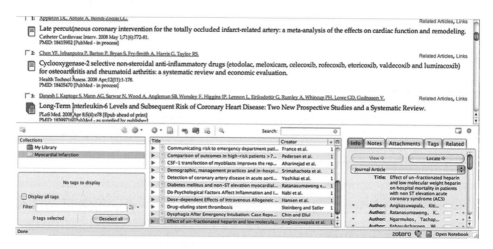

Fig. 4 The Zotero Firefox add-on

appear when Zotero recognizes a Web page, journal article, book, or collection of citations it can capture. For example, if the Web page in your browser is a record for a book on Amazon.com, the icon will look like a book. If it is a PubMed citation, the icon will be a page. If it is a page of PubMed citations (a search), the icon will be a folder. If the icon is a folder, you will get to choose whether to add all citations or to only add selected citations.

Once you've captured a citation, then what? Let's say that you've captured a list of citations from PubMed. Now, you want to add the full text of those articles to the Zotero records. There are several options. One is to add the PDF file of the document as an attachment. The other is to create a snapshot of the Web (HTML) version of the full article.

Here's one relatively simple way to proceed. Zotero automatically captures the snapshot of the PubMed record, listed as an attachment to the citation record. Click on the listing for the snapshot and follow the link to the original Web page – the PubMed record. If you have an institutional affiliation that provides you with access to the full text, or if the article is available for free from the publisher or via PubMed Central, you can usually access the article through the PubMed record (for tips on accessing full-text articles via PubMed, see Sect. 8.5). Once you've accessed the article, select the citation in Zotero. Click on the Attachments tab, click on Add, and select Take Snapshot of Current Page (Fig. 5).

Once you've taken a snapshot, you can view the snapshot to add annotations and highlighting. To open the snapshot, click on the View Snapshot button. Zotero will add a small toolbar to the top of the page with icons allowing you to highlight, dehighlight, and add sticky note annotations to the text (Fig. 6). To add lengthy notes, however, or notes that you may wish to print out later, use the Notes tab in the citation record instead of or in addition to sticky notes.

Major benefit of Zotero over other annotation and note-taking tools is bibliography creation. Zotero provides a plug-in for Word and OpenOffice users that will enable you to add formatted citations directly to a document. At the moment, very few bibliographic styles are available, though National Library of Medicine, Nature, and American Medical Association styles are three options. In addition, you can drag and drop citations into blog posts and online word processing programs like Google Docs.

You can also generate an on-the-fly bibliography. Simply highlight the citations in Zotero, right-click, and select Create Bibliography from Selected Items. You can choose to export the

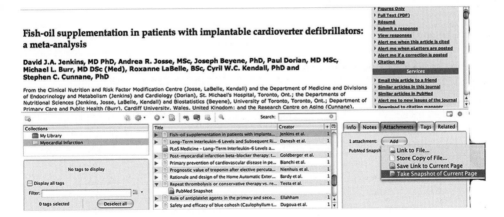

Fig. 5 Adding full text to a Zotero record by taking a snapshot of the current page

19

Data synthesis

Meta-analysis of the 3 trials indicated a nonsignificant relative risk of implantable cardioverter defibril
(RR 0.93, 95% confidence interval [CI] 0.70–1.24, p = 0.63) (Figure 2). None of the 3 studies reported a be
we recalculated relative risk based on the data available from the stu All 3 trials had Jadad scores of 5. e fou
0.56–0.98, p < 0.05).

Fig. 6 Highlighting and sticky notes are helpful Zotero features

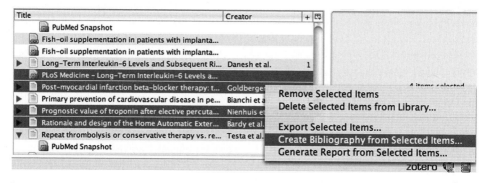

Fig. 7 Creating a bibliography from selected items in Zotero

bibliography as RTF format (word processing) or HTML (Web format), or to copy it to your clipboard (Fig. 7).

19.3.3
Google Notebook

Google Notebook is a Google service that allows you to clip portions of Web pages, bookmark pages, and share the clips and bookmarks you've created with friends. It's not nearly as powerful as the social annotation tools listed above, nor does it have the bibliographic component, but it's a good option for occasional use or if you just don't want to create another Web service account.

Google Notebook requires a browser extension to work correctly. These are available for Firefox 1.5 and higher and Internet Explorer 6

(not Internet Explorer 7). To get started with Google Notebook, go to the Google Notebook site at http://notebook.google.com. You can log in using your Google Account, or if you don't have a Google Account, you can create one.

You'll be prompted to download the appropriate browser extension. You can also visit http://www.google.com/notebook/download/ to install the extension. Once you have the extension installed, you'll see a mini notebook in the bottom bar of your browser. You can click on this at any time to open your mini notebook. Your full-screen notebook, where you can organize your citations, is always online at the main Google Notebook page.

To use Google Notebook, simply highlight the text you want to clip. To send it to your Google Notebook, you can either click on the Clip button in the mini notebook or use the

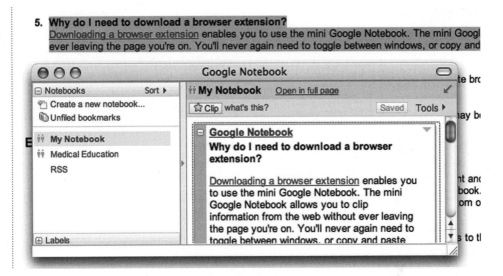

Fig. 8 Using the mini Google Notebook to highlight and clip Web text

right-click context menu to select Note This (Google Notebook). Both will send the clipped text and the link to the Web page to your Google Notebook (Fig. 8).

From the Google Notebook Web site, you can organize your notebook(s) using drag and drop to move clips up and down in the notebook or to another notebook. Create organizational sections and notes using the text box at the top of the notebook. You can also share your notebook with others who have Google Accounts through the Sharing Options link.

19.3.4
Evernote

Evernote (http://www.evernote.com) is a completely different type of tool. Whereas the majority of tools covered in this section were designed to manage and organize Web pages, Evernote is more about organizing your life. You don't just capture Web pages; you capture photos, to do lists, receipts, scribbles, and practically anything you can photograph, scan, or find on the Web. Evernote then takes all your stuff and makes it searchable, even the text on handwritten and photographed notes.

Evernote is in beta, meaning you may not be able to get an invitation immediately. You can sign up for one at the Evernote Web site, however. Evernote is more than just a Web tool; it also works with your cell phone and desktop computer (PC or Mac).

Take the tour of Evernote at http://evernote. com/about/what_is_en/tour/.

19.3.5
Jott

Jott is an audio to text tool designed to help you capture short notes to yourself when you don't have access to a computer – all you need is a phone. Sign up for a Jott account at https://jott. com/register.aspx. You'll need to provide an email address as part of the registration process as well as call Jott from the phone you want to affiliate with your Jott account. Once you've registered, you can send yourself Jotts at any time by calling the phone number Jott provides.

19

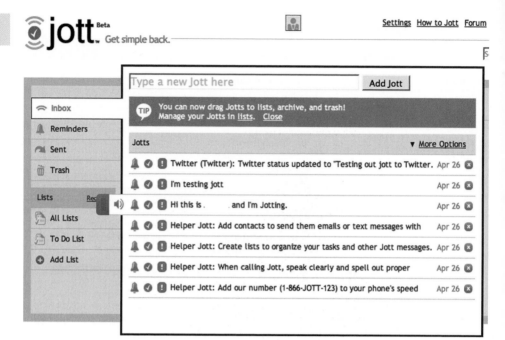

Fig. 9 Jott

Jott is currently only available in the United States and Canada.

Jott lets you set up a connection to other Web services, such as Google Calendar, a WordPress blog, and Facebook. You can send updates to these services just by calling Jott and talking. Jott will convert your voice to text and post your content to your calendar, blog, or other Web service (Fig. 9).

Perhaps, the best feature of Jott is the reminders. If you ever have something you need to remember to pick up or to do, you can Jott it to yourself as a reminder. Jott will send you a text message and email 15 min before the event. You can also Jott to a contact or a group, whether a reminder or just a note. Jotts will be sent as text messages and email.

This is your webcam speaking:
your left optic disc looks glaucomatous ...

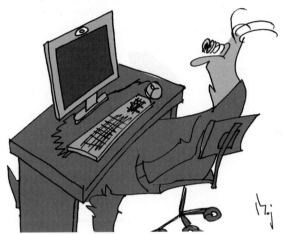

Social Networks

20

Core Messages

> Online social networks let you manage relationships and contact information efficiently.

> Social networks can facilitate the "water cooler consult" on a massive scale.

> Different networks serve different needs and have different revenue models – choose the ones that work best for you and your purposes.

20.1
What's a Social Network?

While a physician might understandably dismiss the idea of joining a social network after having seen the garishness of some MySpace pages and the massive amounts of time that can be wasted in Facebook, we urge physicians to examine several online social networks and try each of them out to see what utility may be found in them.

Social networks are encountered everyday in your analogue life. You know a number of people and each of them knows a number of people. If you draw a line between each person and the people they know, you'll start to see patterns emerge in the spider web of lines produced. The problem is that, even if you had the time to draw such a thorough map of relationships between everyone you know, you don't have the knowledge. Online social networks are one way to map the complex Web of interconnection between people, because they provide an efficient way to construct and manage the extraordinarily complex map of relationships you work with everyday. For many, online social networks replace the Rolodex or address book.

Online social networks for physicians hold a special appeal, however, because they allow the practice of the "water cooler consult" on a massive scale and despite great potential geographic distance. What if you need a quick opinion from an experienced gastroenterologist but the one you usually would go to is out of town and unreachable? Wouldn't it be nice to put your question to a group of credentialed physicians in that specialty?

Social networks can act as filters for the massive amount of new clinical information produced everyday. Rather than reading every new article in your field, you might instead use a physicians' social network to see what your peers may have thought about a particular article. If, for instance, several physicians whose judgment you trust use the social network to indicate that they found a particular article not worth the time it took to read, you may decide to not invest

M. Rethlefsen et al., *Internet Cool Tools for Physicians*
© Springer-Verlag Berlin Heidelberg 2009

20

the time reading it yourself. If several of your peers indicate that a particular article is particularly good, you might want to make a point of setting aside the time to read it carefully.

20.2
Which Social Networks Should I Consider Joining?

There's no shortage of options – here are just a few.

20.2.1
LinkedIn (http://www.linkedin.com/)

LinkedIn is promoted as a social network for professionals. Unlike Facebook, there aren't any cute virtual gifts or games here. LinkedIn is a serious site where users post all their professional information, note their relationships with colleagues and other professional contacts, meet new people through their contacts, or even write testimonials in which they recommend a contact or a contact's work. LinkedIn's users are from all professions, but there's no doubt that a good number of physicians are members of LinkedIn (Fig. 1).

20.2.2
Sermo (http://www.sermo.com/)

In May 2007, the American Medical Association formed an official partnership with Sermo, an online social network for doctors. At the time of this writing, Sermo is probably the most popular US-based online social network for physicians

with more than 65,000 members. Sermo is adamant that members must be credentialed physicians and has a proprietary method for vetting members as licensed physicians when they sign up for free membership (Fig. 2).

While Sermo (its name taken from the Latin word for "conversation") is free for physicians to use, Sermo's revenue model has caused concern in some quarters. Sermo describes its model as "one of information arbitrage." Many organizations (including financial institutions, regulatory bodies, specialty societies, pharmaceutical manufacturers, and others) pay a premium to Sermo for the right to access the conversations that physicians have on Sermo. Physicians should consider this before deciding to join Sermo and make certain that they are comfortable with this arrangement. While it isn't uncommon on the Web to trade personal information (usually for marketing purposes) in exchange for services, Sermo's extension of this model is a new sort of idea that may or may not take off.

For details on Sermo's revenue model, see notes from their Frequently Asked Questions at http://www.sermo.com/about/faqs#money.

20.2.3
Ozmosis (http://www.ozmosis.com/)

Ozmosis is another online social network intended for the exclusive use of physicians. New members are automatically screened and credentialed when they join Ozmosis and are required to use their real names, not aliases or User IDs. This helps to assure all users of Ozmosis that the opinions they are getting from other users are from credentialed physicians whose names are attached to what they write. This level of accountability is intended

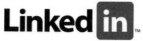
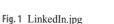

Fig. 1 LinkedIn.jpg

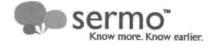

Fig. 2 Sermo.jpg

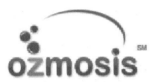

Fig. 3 Ozmosis.jpg

to keep the quality of discourse on Ozmosis high (Fig. 3).

Ozmosis allows you to add other users to your "trusted" group and judge the quality of advice you may get from the friend of a friend by seeing how many people you trust also trust the giver of advice. Ozmosis does not disclose content created by users to third parties and does not contain advertising, but it does allow members to "opt-in" to "sponsored areas."

20.2.4
Variations on a Theme

There are a number of other general social networks for physicians that appear to be variations on a theme.

Physicians in the United Kingdom will want to take a look at Doctors.net.uk (http://www.doctors.net.uk/), which, at the time of this writing, has about 155,000 physician members from the UK.

Networks like MedicSpeak (http://www.medicspeak.com/), SocialMD (http://www.socialmd.com/), DoctorsHangout (http://doctorshangout.com/) and TiroMed (http://www.tiromed.com/) open their doors not only to physicians but also to medical students. Medical students who join may find not only support from their contemporaries, but also mentoring from and connections with physicians working in the specialties the students

hope to pursue. Healtheva (http://www.healtheva.com/) welcomes physicians, researchers, residents, interns, and medical students. Prometeo (http://www.prometeonetwork.com/) is for both physicians and researchers in the life sciences.

RelaxDoc (http://www.relaxdoc.com/), Doctor Networking (http://www.doctornetworking.com/), and Clinical Village (http://clinicalvillage.com/) are three other networks for physicians that don't seem to have significantly distinguished themselves from the pack.

20.2.5
Specialty Networks

Another whole category of online social networks are those built around a particular specialty. RadRounds (http://www.radrounds.com/) is a social network for radiologists and Syndicom-SpineConnect (http://www.syndicom.com/spineconnect/) is an online social network exclusively for spine surgeons. We suspect that social networks revolving around a particular specialty will be a growing trend and wouldn't be at all surprised if, in the not terribly distant future, most professional associations had their own online social networks.

20.3
Ethics

When sharing information about or seeking advice on a particular patient in a social network or any online forum, be sure to protect the patient's privacy to the same degree you would if you were writing up the case for publication.

Printing: Krips bv, Meppel, The Netherlands
Binding: Stürtz, Würzburg, Germany